The Organic PSYCHOSES

PSYCHOSES due to physical disturbances involving the brain are common and can complicate a bewildering variety of illnesses. Patients with such disorders may be encountered in general practice, emergency wards, medical services, on the surgical wards post-operatively as well as in psychiatric units of general hospitals, psychiatric clinics and of course in mental hospitals. A specialist in psychiatry and a specialist in internal medicine have collaborated to fill an important gap in medical literature of practical value to the physician. Throughout the book the needs of doctors who are responsible for such patients has been kept in mind. In this well-organized, concise monograph the organic psychoses are classified in a comprehensive manner which can be easily applied to clinical cases. The chief diagnostic features of the various organic syndromes have been presented, together with full references to the clinical literature. The diagnostic approach to the various clinical problems has been considered and illustrated by a group of case histories. As teachers, the authors have become aware of the need for a clarification of this complicated area of medicine in order that the practitioner, postgraduate physician, interne, and undergraduate student may have a ready guide to aid him in the diagnosis of these complicated disorders. Many doctors in a number of branches of medical practice will find this a handy, useful book to own.

JOHN G. DEWAN, M.A., M.D., PH.D. CANTAB., D.P.M. ENG., F.R.C.P. (C), F.A.P.A., F.A.C.P., is Associate Professor of Psychiatry, University of Toronto, and Director of the Out-Patient Department, Toronto Psychiatric Hospital. He was formerly a Beit Memorial Research Fellow, University of Cambridge.

WILLIAM B. SPAULDING, M.D., F.R.C.P. (C), is Associate Professor of Medicine, and Associate, Department of Psychiatry, University of Toronto. He is Physician in charge of the Medical Out-Patient Department, Toronto General Hospital. Dr. Spaulding was a Markle Scholar, 1951-1956.

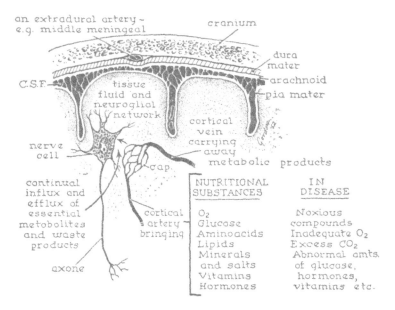

Diagrammatic representation of the cerebral neurone and its milieu

THE
ORGANIC PSYCHOSES

A Guide to Diagnosis

by

JOHN G. DEWAN

M.A., M.D., Ph.D. Cantab.,
D.P.M. Eng., F.R.C.P.(C), F.A.C.P., F.A.P.A.

Associate Professor of Psychiatry, University of Toronto
Director Out-Patient Department,
Toronto Psychiatric Hospital
Formerly Beit Memorial Research Fellow,
University of Cambridge

and

WILLIAM B. SPAULDING

M.D., F.R.C.P.(C)

Associate Professor of Medicine, and Associate, Department of
Psychiatry, University of Toronto
Physician in charge of Medical Out-Patient Department,
Toronto General Hospital
Formerly Markle Scholar

UNIVERSITY OF TORONTO PRESS, 1958

FOREWORD

This monograph on "The Organic Psychoses" arose out of the authors' experiences with patients admitted from the community to either a psychiatric hospital or a general hospital. A not inconsiderable number showed presumptive evidence of an organic mental state: some were confused and disturbing; others were bemused and inert. Whether or not the difficulties of home management had decided the admission it was often evident that the diagnostic problem had been accorded scant attention.

The general psychiatric diagnosis was not usually obscure: manifestations of the more acute or more chronic organic psychoses are, in the main, clearly recognizable. The pathological diagnosis, the finding of a principal physical cause in the particular instance, was the major difficulty for the receiving physicians. A mesh of systemic relationships had to be teased out quickly in orderly fashion. Orderliness of investigation became the core of concern.

Recognizing the many origins of upset and the wide range of dislocating agents, the authors took as their point of reference the cell body of the cerebral neurone. From this focus they examined, sector by sector, the possible areas of disturbance, each considered in turn, until evidence of a noxious process was shown conclusively. Clearly the diagnostic method allows both a priority scanning of the common causes and, by extension in any sector, a review of the rarer upsets.

It is astonishing, particularly when cellular and chemical pathology are in rapid advance, that the field of the organic psychoses has been relatively neglected in practice. Internists seem to avoid a purposeful investigation of cases presenting as psychosis: psychiatrists oftentimes lack the necessary techniques and facilities. Good clinical and laboratory organizations are necessary: their warranty is the saving of life and, even more, the not infrequent restoration of healthy living where previously a frantic violence or dazed stupor had raised the worst fears of unrelieved insanity.

The restoration process goes beyond the finding of physical causes and their control by appropriate physical measures. Opportunities for both psychological and social treatment offer themselves continuously, the former where a personal pattern of living has initiated the physical insult—the latter where adjustments to a residual disability or to the social effects of the acute illness have to be faced.

The organic psychoses, while challenging all the medical disciplines, comprise a field for integrated study, particularly by the pathologist, the internist, and the psychiatrist. Sometimes, in clinical psychiatric practice, it appears as if the problems of the organic psychoses have been "given up": rather is the need that they be "taken up."

Over and above their contribution to method, the authors have invited a renewed, enthusiastic interest in one of the most difficult territories of medical exploration and treatment responsibility.

ALDWYN STOKES
Professor and Head of the
Department of Psychiatry
University of Toronto

PREFACE

The decision to write this book arose out of the need of resident doctors in general and psychiatric hospitals in our community for a brief and systematic guide to the diagnosis of organic psychoses. It is reasonable to suppose that the same need exists elsewhere and is not, by any means, confined to hospital residents. The diagnostic problems in the field of organic mental illness are fundamentally similar the world over and may be encountered by doctors anywhere who are confronted with patients having mental symptoms. We believe the physician who attempts to unravel such problems will find it helpful to have, as part of his diagnostic equipment, an orderly guide to the collection of information and a systematic approach to the analysis of the data. We think there is a place for a small monograph which is not intended to be an encyclopaedic textbook but rather presents the essentials of the subject with a view to simplifying the problems of diagnosis for the practising physician as well as for the resident doctor.

It is generally understood that in every case of mental illness the possibility of a contributing physical factor should be kept in mind. The frequency with which the physical factor is overlooked and the tendency to uncertainty (sometimes unavoidable) in understanding the causation of mental disorders have been an additional reason for writing this guide to the diagnosis of organic mental illness.

It should be stated at the beginning that, although the importance of organic factors is being stressed, there is no intention of minimizing the role of psychological and social forces in the maintenance of mental health or the genesis of mental ill health. Furthermore, while physical factors may be of prime importance in the aetiology of an organic psychosis, one should not be surprised that the general clinical picture may also be determined by the personality make-up of the particular patient who is ill. Indeed, in some cases in the early stages of the illness, or when the physical component is of relatively minor significance, the mental picture may be that of a so-called functional illness: for example, anxiety state, depression, schizophrenia or paranoid reaction. In such cases, to avoid the pitfall of a mistaken diagnosis, the physician must be alert to the possibility of an operating organic factor and be aware of the clinical symptoms and signs of organic psychosis, as well as the laboratory aids at his disposal.

We are using the term organic psychosis (organic syndrome; organic psychiatric disorder) with reference to any mental illness in which a physical (organic) factor, disturbing the functioning of brain tissue, is playing a sufficient role to be of major importance in causing the breakdown. In most instances the physical factor eventually contributes to the psychiatric picture itself by giving rise to delirium or dementia. The organic factor may be one of many possible physical and chemical agents or processes which impair the functioning of the brain cells. The resultant syndromes have certain characteristics which will be described later in the text. The impairment of the functioning of cerebral tissue in some cases may be reversible, in others permanent and not changing or progressive.

With these principles in mind we have attempted in Parts I and II to describe briefly and systematically the organic mental illnesses from an aetiological standpoint, emphasizing distinguishing features, both clinical and laboratory. The information in these sections is designed to provide an orderly minimum of facts which the physician should have in mind before dealing with the clinical problems. Some may object that the descriptions of diseases are too sketchy. However, we have chosen to provide a large-scale map of this area of medicine rather than a detailed, finely drawn diagram. Therefore lengthy descriptions and discussions of pathology or treatment which can be found in comprehensive textbooks have been deliberately avoided. It is taken for granted that the reader is reasonably well grounded in the elements of psychiatry and medicine. In order to make the book more useful a considerable number of clinically oriented references have been included. These can be consulted to provide the details which one so often wishes to know in studying individual patients. The references are drawn, for the most part, from journals and books written in English and available in most medical libraries. Part III is devoted to the strictly practical approach to individual cases, illustrating the variety of problems which may be encountered and indicating the steps which lead to final diagnosis.

The diagnostic problems discussed are encountered not only by internists and psychiatrists but also by general practitioners, neurologists, neurosurgeons and other specialists. To all doctors who, like ourselves, have been and still are bewildered by the difficulties in this branch of medicine, we address this book in the hope that it may prove useful. In addition, nurses, social workers and psychologists working in the field of psychological medicine may find that the book increases their understanding of the nature and manifestations of organic brain disease.

The authors owe a debt of thanks to many helpful persons. In particular we should like to mention Miss Elizabeth Wright, Miss F. McKinley, Miss J. H. Rawkins, Mrs. B. W. Higgs, Mrs. B. Wilshire and Mrs. D. Schurman who have handled the secretarial duties so ably. Miss Houston, of the staff of the University of Toronto Press, has been patient and given much helpful advice in the preparation of the manuscript. Dr. E. A. Linell, Professor Emeritus of Neuropathology at the University of Toronto, has been most generous in allowing us free access to his excellent autopsy reports and has discussed with us several of the cases in detail. The case histories are based on the work of too many doctors to name individually, but we should like to mention the post-graduate physicians who have worked in the organic psychosis unit at the Toronto Psychiatric Hospital in the last few years: Doctors L. Bow, D. E. Zarfas, S. Feldman, R. Pos and W. Woodruff. We owe special thanks to Professor A. B. Stokes who has encouraged us throughout the preparation of the book.

Toronto   J. G. D.
July 1958   W. B. S.

CONTENTS

PART I

The Causative Factors of the Organic Psychoses

CHAPTER I

The Cerebral Cell as a Focal Point

Consideration of the physical agents and mechanisms which may produce organic psychoses should be undertaken on the basis of brain physiology. Thinking, feeling and general behaviour are dependent ultimately on body functioning, especially on that of the central nervous system, a cellular tissue having as its unit the neurone or nerve cell. Since the cerebral neurone plays a fundamental role in psychic experience and may be influenced by many physico-chemical factors, it is well to focus attention on this cell and its immediate environment.

Developmentally, these cerebral cells require certain conditions for growth. The germ plasm from which they originate by ectodermal differentiation must be healthy, otherwise anomalies of development—for example, agenesis or hypogenesis—may occur, with resultant impaired cerebral functioning. During intra-uterine life and the remainder of the growing period, the hormonal control must be correctly balanced. In the case of cretinism, due to a deficiency in the production of thyroid hormone, normal maturation of the nervous system fails to occur. The nutritive requirements include an adequate supply of lipids for the production of lecithin, sphingomyelin and cerebroside to ensure the healthy development of the nerve cells, including their myelin sheaths. Amino acids must be available for the synthesis of nucleoproteins, cytoplasmic proteins, and enzymes—the cellular catalysts. Carbohydrates are especially essential for the energy yielding mechanisms of the cell. Oxygen, minerals, salts, vitamins and water are a few of the many chemical substances necessary. Although the nervous system may have developed normally, the neurones are vulnerable to deleterious physical and chemical influences of many different types throughout the lifetime of the organism. Once lethally injured, they cannot be replaced by the multiplication of remaining neurones. However, the tremendous reserve and adaptability of uninjured brain tissues compensates to an amazing degree in many instances.

Certain factors in the environment of nerve cells are of profound importance. The neurones are sensitive to disturbances of intracranial mechanics. It can be readily appreciated that distortion of the neurones, either by traction, as in the case of shrinking scar tissue, or by pressure from a space-occupying lesion, will interfere with the continuous, healthy cellular activity. Between the neurones and neuroglial cells lies a milieu, the tissue fluid. In addition to its supportive function, this milieu provides a medium for the passage of oxygen, carbohydrate, lipids, amino acids, minerals, hormones, vitamins, etc. from the capillaries to the nerve cells. The amounts of water, salt and protein are balanced within narrow physiological limits in the tissue fluid to ensure proper hydration of the nerve cells, passage of electrolytes such as potassium, magnesium and chloride ions across the cell membranes, and maintenance of normal osmotic pressure in cells, tissue fluids and blood. Products of tissue metabolism diffuse through the tissue fluid in the reverse direction, from neurone to capillaries and venous system. The cell also has communication with the cerebrospinal fluid by way of the perineuronal space. The cell is sensitive to any alteration in the concentration of normal constituents of the extracellular fluid, and is affected by the presence of chemical substances foreign to its immediate environment, whether derived from disordered metabolism in the body or introduced from the organism's external environment.

Most, if not all, of the myriad chemical reactions in the cell are catalysed by enzymes. These organic catalysts are frequently proteins combined with simpler substances, the prosthetic groups. Some of these prosthetic groups contain members of the vitamin B-complex. As an example, the pyrophosphoric ester of thiamine (Vitamin B_1) is the prosthetic group of carboxylase, the enzyme which catalyses the metabolism of pyruvic acid. A deficiency of thiamine results in diminished oxidation of pyruvic acid, thus producing disordered functioning of the nerve cell and other cells of the body, utlimately reflected in the clinical states, Korsakoff's syndrome, Wernicke's encephalopathy and beriberi. A defect in the chemical structure of an enzyme, or its absence, also may lead to abnormal metabolism in the cell. Phenylpyruvic oligophrenia is a clinical disorder thought to be due to such a mechanism. It is considered the result of a homozygous genetic abnormality that affects an enzyme which normally catalyses the conversion of the amino acid phenylalanine to tyrosine. As a result of the enzymatic defect, phenylpyruvic acid accumulates in the tissues and the urine. The potency of hormones in minute amounts suggests the likelihood that they, too, are intimately involved in enzyme systems. Certain metals also are integral units of the cell's catalytic organization. For example, cobalt has been demonstrated within the molecule vitamin B_{12} (cyanocobolamin), iron in cytochrome and cytochrome oxidase, copper in ceruloplasmin. Any abnormality in the structure or quantity of such fundamental substances can disturb the delicate balance of the interrelated chemical mechanisms of the cells of the brain and other tissues, with far-reaching disorder of the functioning of the organism. Some chemical substances, arising from a metabolic defect either within the body or from the environment, may inhibit temporarily or alter permanently the enzymes of the cell. A number of these substances, because of their similarity in chemical structure to the normal substrates in the cell, combine with enzymes preventing them from activating the metabolites. Certain drugs and chemical toxins are thought to be functioning in this manner as competitors or antimetabolites, thus interfering with cellular metabolism. (Indeed, it has been postulated that even functional mental illnesses, such as schizophrenia, may be due primarily to such mechanisms resulting from a fault in the metabolism of the cells.)

With the neurone and its milieu (see frontispiece) as our focus, we can now turn to a detailed consideration of the many factors that may disturb nerve cell functioning. This approach forms a sound basis for an aetiological classification of organic psychoses.

REFERENCE

HIMWICH, H. E.: Thought processes as related to brain metabolism in certain abnormal conditions, J. Nerv. & Ment. Dis. 114:450, Nov. 1951.

CHAPTER II

An Aetiological Classification
of Organic Psychoses

A fairly comprehensive list of the causes of organic psychoses will be presented in this chapter. Many of the diseases listed in the classification are rare, but rare conditions cannot be diagnosed unless one is familiar with such possibilities. Furthermore, it may be important to make a comprehensive differential diagnosis early in the illness and then narrow the number of diagnostic possibilities down as quickly as possible by appropriate investigation. There are two reasons for attempting to reach a firm diagnosis with the least possible delay. Firstly, in the case of some infections, drug intoxications and metabolic disturbances, laboratory tests of prime diagnostic importance may be negative unless they are carried out in the first days of the illness. Secondly, in remediable conditions such as bacterial meningitis or subdural haematoma, the earlier treatment is begun, the better will be the prognosis.

Although an attempt has been made to construct a consistent classification based on physico-chemical factors affecting cerebral cells, this goal cannot be completely attained because of the still limited knowledge of cellular physiology and our ignorance concerning the way in which certain disease states are produced. Furthermore, a deficiency or excess of a hormone, an electrolyte or certain elements may result in widespread dislocation of the internal chemical environment of the body, and it is difficult to know whether the resulting mental disorder is due to the original metabolic defect or due to the secondary biochemical disturbances or indeed due to all of these factors. For example, we have classified mental disorders associated with Addison's disease under hypofunction of the adrenal cortex. These disorders, however, may not be due, at least entirely, to the effect of decreased concentrations of adrenal steroids on the functioning of cerebral cells, but may be the result, in part at least, of an accompanying hypoglycaemia, low concentrations of sodium and chloride ion, high levels of potassium, or water disturbance. Indeed, correction of some of these secondary disorders without any attention to the low level of adrenal cortical hormone may result in improved physical and mental functioning.

In addition to these reservations, one must keep in mind the basic principle of multiple aetiology. Organic factors are operating synergistically with social and psychological stresses in a particular constitution, all factors contributing in varying degrees to the genesis of the breakdown and to the presenting clinical picture. (For completeness, we have included in the classification several examples of mental deficiency which will receive little consideration in the text because mental deficiency is not generally included in the organic psychoses.)

1. METABOLIC DISORDERS (including disturbed supply of nutriment and other substances essential for metabolism of cerebral cells)
(a) *Carbohydrate*
   Hypoglycaemia
   (i) Functional
   (ii) Secondary to:
      insulin therapy
      islet cell adenoma
      anterior pituitary insufficiency
      adrenal insufficiency
      severe liver disease
   (Hyperglycaemia—there is no definite evidence that a high glucose level per se causes psychoses)

(*b*) *Fat*
  (i) Amaurotic family idiocy (Tay Sach's disease: cere-
      bromacular degeneration—a lipid disorder confined to
      the central nervous system)
  (ii) Hand-Schüller-Christian disease (a disorder of choles-
       terol metabolism usually resulting in widespread
       lesions)
(*c*) *Protein and Amino Acids*
  Phenylpyruvic oligophrenia (defect in the metabolism of
  the aromatic amino acid phenylalanine)
(*d*) *Vitamin Deficiency*
  (i) Thiamine (Vitamin B_1: aneurin)
      Korsakoff's syndrome
      Wernicke's encephalopathy
      Beriberi
  (ii) Nicotinic acid (niacin)
       Pellagra
  (iii) Vitamin B_{12}
        Pernicious anaemia with subacute combined de-
        generation
(*e*) *Minerals*
  (i) Iron deficiency (the accompanying haemoglobin de-
      ficiency may impair cerebral oxidations)
  (ii) Calcium deficiency (e.g. in hypoparathyroidism)
  (iii) Calcium excess (e.g. in hyperparathyroidism)
  (iv) Disordered copper metabolism (e.g. Wilson's disease:
       hepato-lenticular degeneration)
  (v) Others (e.g. magnesium deficiency)
(*f*) *Porphyrins* (e.g. porphyria)
(*g*) *Electrolytes*
  For example:
  (i) Low blood sodium and chloride with high blood po-
      tassium (the pattern in adrenal cortical insufficiency)
  (ii) High blood sodium, low potassium and low chloride
       (the pattern in adrenal cortical hyperfunction)

(*h*) *Acid Base Balance* (pH)
Acidosis and Alkalosis
(*i*) *Water*
Dehydration with an associated electrolyte upset
(*j*) *Hormones*
(i) Pituitary
Anterior pituitary insufficiency (Simmond's disease)
(ii) Adrenal
Adrenal cortical insufficiency (Addison's disease)
Adrenal cortical hyperfunction (Cushing's syndrome)
(iii) Thyroid
Hyperthyroidism (Grave's disease—the syndrome of exophthalmos and thyrotoxicosis)
Hypothyroidism (cretinism; myxoedema)
(iv) Parathyroid
Hyperparathyroidism
Hypoparathyroidism
(v) Pancreas
Hyperinsulinism
(*k*) *Oxygen*
Decreased supply of oxygen to cerebral cells may be due to:
(i) Inadequate oxygen in the atmosphere
(ii) Pulmonary disease and impaired pulmonary circulation
(iii) Deficient carrying power of the blood, e.g. carbon monoxide poisoning or severe anaemia
(iv) Slowing or cessation of blood flow as found in profound shock
(v) Intracellular interference with normal oxygen utilization and oxidative processes (e.g. due to drugs)

2. DISORDERED BLOOD SUPPLY OF CEREBRAL CELLS
(*a*) Cerebral Atherosclerosis

(b) Thrombosis
(c) Haemorrhage
(d) Embolism
(e) Slowing of Blood Flow (e.g. cardiac failure)
(f) Less Common Types of Vascular Disease (e.g. poly-
     areritis nodosa, disseminated lupus erythematosus,
     temporal arteritis)

3. MECHANICAL STRESSES INTERFERING WITH CEREBRAL
   FUNCTIONING
   (a) Space-occupying Lesions (e.g. tumour, haematoma,
        abscess)
   (b) Obstruction to Cerebrospinal Fluid Circulation
   (c) Trauma

4. INFECTIONS
   (a) *Primarily Affecting the Central Nervous System*
        (i) Meningitis due to pyogenic bacteria, tubercle bacilli
             or treponema pallidum
        (ii) Encephalitis due to viruses, including those causing
             mumps and measles
        (iii) General paralysis of the insane (general paresis)
   (b) *Other Infections Sometimes Producing Mental Symptoms*
        (e.g. typhoid fever, pneumococcal pneumonia, cysti-
        cercosis)

5. INTOXICATIONS
   (a) *Exogenous*
        (i) Medication
             (1) Sedatives (e.g. bromides, barbiturates)
             (2) Stimulants (e.g. benzedrine)
             (3) Chemotherapeutic and antibiotic agents (e.g.
                  sulpha drugs, arsenicals, atabrine, penicillin)
             (4) Hormones (e.g. adrenocorticotrophic hormone,
                  cortisone, insulin, thyroid)

(5) Hypotensor drugs (e.g. thiocyanate, reserpine)
(6) Miscellaneous (e.g. antihistaminic drugs)
(ii) Self Administered
    (1) Alcohol
        Acute intoxication
        Delirium tremens
        Hallucinosis
        Korsakoff's syndrome
        Dementia
    (2) Others (e.g. cocaine, marihuana)
(iii) Occupational (e.g. lead, manganese, methyl chloride, carbon disulphide)
(b) *Endogenous*
    (e.g. uraemia, hepatic failure)

6. DEGENERATIONS OF CEREBRAL TISSUE
    Huntington's chorea
    Alzheimer's disease
    Pick's disease
    Senile atrophy
    Disseminated sclerosis
    Schilder's disease
    Tuberous sclerosis (epiloia)
    Friedreich's ataxia
        The causes of these diseases are unknown.

7. PAROXYSMAL CEREBRAL DYSRYTHMIAS (the epilepsies; epilepsy)
    Psychomotor attacks and post-convulsive psychotic episodes occur in epilepsy:
(a) *Secondary to Physical Factors* (many of which are included in this classification of organic psychosis)
(b) *Idiopathic*

PART II

Clinical Features

INTRODUCTION

Generally speaking, one can divide the clinical patterns into two broad groups: (*a*) delirious states and (*b*) dementia. Both groups may also exhibit mood and thought disorders such as mania, depression, paranoid thinking. However, not all patients suffering from an organic psychosis have obvious symptoms of dementia or delirium. The mental states may be very similar to those of "functional" psychoses such as schizophrenia or paranoia. Careful clinical examination commonly reveals "organic" mental symptoms (see Clinical Investigative Approach, p. 75).

Usually the aetiology of an organic psychosis cannot be deduced from the particular mental picture. Because the mental status is not of specific help in the differential diagnosis of the organic lesion, no attempt has been made to describe the varied psychotic syndromes which may occur in a given type of organic psychosis. The following clinical descriptions will therefore be found lacking in this regard. If the reader will study the case reports presented in later chapters, he will soon appreciate the wide variations in mental symptomatology.

CHAPTER III

Metabolic Disorders

(Including disturbed supply of nutriment and other substances
essential for the metabolism of cerebral cells)

(*a*) *Carbohydrate*

In conformity with the classification of causes, we will
begin the consideration of metabolic disorders by discussing
the chief diagnostic features of *hypoglycaemia*. The settings
in which hypoglycaemia occurs may be divided into functional
and secondary. Patients with functional hypoglycaemia frequently are anxious and under psychological stress. In these
patients the physiological defect responsible for the fall in
blood sugar is not known. The chief causes of secondary
hypoglycaemia are insulin excess, either exogenous or endogenous, diffuse hepatic disease and insufficiency of the anterior
pituitary or adrenal glands.

Acute episodes. Cerebral and autonomic dysfunction
account for the outstanding clinical manifestations accompanying marked hypoglycaemia regardless of its cause. Frequently,
the mental state is one of mild anxiety or a slight degree of
confusion, but occasionally there is a more marked disturbance
occurring transiently, with the fairly rapid appearance of confusion, restlessness, noisiness and a maniacal state often like
that of acute alcoholic intoxication. Convulsions and coma
are occasionally seen. There may be focal disorders—paraesthesias or transient paralyses, for example. The autonomic
response closely resembles the reaction to a large dose of
adrenaline and has many features of the acute anxiety state.
Common symptoms are: marked sweating, tremulousness,
palpitation, headache, and hunger feelings or "gone" feelings
in the epigastrium.

The periodicity of the symptoms is of prime diagnostic importance. In functional hypoglycaemia the episodes occur two to four hours after a meal, particularly one rich in carbohydrate. Interestingly enough, prolonged fasting will not bring on an attack. The regulatory mechanisms for blood sugar control function adequately in the fasting state, but there is an over-response to the rise in blood sugar which follows carbohydrate intake. Where hypoglycaemia is secondary to some other cause, such as adrenal cortical insufficiency or islet cell adenoma producing an excess of insulin, the episodes occur following a prolonged fast. In either functional or secondary hypoglycaemia the taking of carbohydrate promptly relieves the symptoms.

The laboratory findings are quite distinctive. The blood sugar is always below 70 mg. per 100 ml. during an attack. A glucose tolerance test carried on for five or six hours may clarify the diagnosis in difficult cases. In patients with functional hypoglycaemia the test will commonly reveal: a normal or mildly depressed fasting blood sugar, a curve with the lowest blood sugar two to four hours after the administration of glucose and a tendency for the blood sugar to return to normal toward the end of the test without the administration of food or glucose. The same test in the patient with hyperinsulinism due to a pancreatic adenoma will often reveal: a fasting blood sugar of about 40 to 60 mg. per 100 ml., then a normal or exaggerated rise, followed by a rather sharp fall to about 40 mg. per 100 ml. three hours or more after the glucose. In the four to six hour interval there is no spontaneous rise to normal fasting levels.

Chronic sequelae (to severe prolonged hypoglycaemia). In some patients with severe, acute adrenal cortical insufficiency, or individuals receiving or manufacturing too much insulin, profound dementia may ensue. Brain metabolism is singularly dependent on oxygen and glucose. If either or both are lacking, cells degenerate, first those of the cortex, then basal ganglia and brain stem. The blood sugar estimation is not helpful after prolonged hypoglycaemia has been corrected, because it will be normal despite the persistence of the dementia.

(b) Fat

(i) Amaurotic family idiocy

This is a rare familial disease affecting infants, predominantly but not exclusively Hebrew. Its main features are severe mental deficiency, blindness, presence of a cherry-red macular spot on retinal examination, paralysis of all four limbs and a uniformly fatal outcome before age two. The abnormal accumulation of a lipid substance in the brain is thought to be responsible for the widespread cerebral atrophy. The lipid is composed of a cerebroside (containing sphingosine, fatty acid and galactose), plus neuramic acid (a nitrogen containing organic acid).

There is a juvenile form of the same disease which may have its onset up to as late as age twenty-five. In this form of the disease, the course is more prolonged.

(ii) Hand-Schüller-Christian disease

This is a rare disorder of childhood in which xanthomatous lesions destroy bones, particularly those of the skull. Cholesterol is found in the lesions in large amounts. Diabetes insipidus due to pituitary destruction, exophthalmos due to masses arising in the orbital walls and retardation of growth are the main clinical findings. Mental development may be impaired.

(c) Protein and Amino Acids

Phenylpyruvic oligophrenia. This disease results in mental deficiency plus the urinary excretion of phenylpyruvic acid, an abnormal excretion product of phenylalanine metabolism. The urine turns dark green when ferric chloride solution is added (ee technical appendix p. 160). The condition has been found in less than one per cent of mental defectives surveyed in large institutions. It is familial and tends to occur in blond, fair-skinned individuals. Some patients have involvement of the extra-pyramidal system, resulting in rigidity and hypertonicity.

(d) *Vitamin Deficiency*

From a clinical standpoint, vitamin deficiencies are nearly always multiple, and often associated with protein deficit. It is obvious that a patient (such as a chronic alcoholic or a food faddist) who is eating a nutritionally inadequate diet will lack more than one vitamin. Furthermore, patients with a marked decrease in the absorptive surface of the bowel resulting from various types of gastro-intestinal disease, or from surgical removal or short-circuiting of portions of their gastro-intestinal tract, will have difficulty in absorbing not one but several essential foodstuffs.

In certain parts of the world where malnutrition is common, vitamin B deficiency is said to be a fairly frequent cause of mental illness, particularly in elderly patients. Some authors describe clinical states indistinguishable from psychoneuroses, but relieved by the administration of vitamin B complex. A type of encephalopathy, usually fatal unless treated with nicotinic acid, has been reported. Such conditions are rare in countries with high standards of nutrition but should be kept in mind.

(i) *Thiamine deficiency*

In Canada, the most common setting for this condition is severe, prolonged alcoholism. In some patients the mental symptoms are very distinctive. When severe loss of memory for recent events occurs in conjunction with striking confabulation, the term Korsakoff's syndrome applies. Brain stem signs are frequently seen and when associated with changes in consciousness and a confusional state the term Wernicke's syndrome is used. Brain stem signs include pupillary changes (inequality, loss of reaction to light), extra-ocular muscle palsies and nystagmus; severe ataxia and slurred, dysarthric speech are commonly present. These abnormalities fluctuate rapidly over a period of hours or days. In thiamine deficiency there is always the danger of permanent damage to the central nervous system with residual dementia, not infrequently accompanied by confabulation. In some instances the mental state may deteriorate from one of delirium to coma; in neglected or unrecognized cases death may occur.

Thiamine deficiency also causes heart disease with certain features found in "high-output failure": tachycardia, high pulse pressure, capillary pulsation and bounding pulse, warm, red extremities and congestive failure. The heart becomes dilated. Tachycardia plus low voltage are the main electrocardiographic abnormalities. Peripheral oedema, without cardiac failure, is seen in some patients. Peripheral neuritis is commonly present, with striking tenderness of the muscles of the legs as a feature.

Laboratory confirmation: the pyruvic acid blood levels following glucose ingestion rise sharply and do not fall in several hours, as is the case in normal subjects. Thiamine lack prevents the breakdown of pyruvic acid to carbon dioxide and water.

(ii) *Nicotinic acid deficiency*
The following are the more common clinical features: the skin becomes photosensitive with the result that exposed areas redden, blister and tan. The end stage of the dermatitis is thickening and pigmentation of the face, neck, forearms and hands. Mucous membrane involvement gives rise to a sore, smooth, red tongue, diarrhoea and an irritative, itching vaginal discharge. Mental delirium and deterioration may occur.

Almost always, signs of other vitamin deficiencies may be found, such as the magenta tongue and fissuring of the angles of the lips found in riboflavin lack.

(iii) *Vitamin B$_{12}$ deficiency*

The disease produced is pernicious anaemia. The anaemia is hyperchromic and macrocytic, with a colour index greater than 1. When severe, the anaemia may be accompanied by anorexia, weakness, loss of weight, breathlessness and a yellowish pallor of the skin.

Mucosal change results in an intermittently sore, strikingly smooth and clean tongue, free from papillae and débris. Most, but not all, patients have such an abnormality of their tongues. The gastric mucosa always atrophies so that, even after histamine injection, there will be no free hydrochloric acid in the gastric contents. Patients may have troublesome diarrhoea.

Neurological and psychiatric disorders may be prominent and, on rare occasions, exist in the absence of anaemia. Peripheral neuritis, manifested by numbness and tingling in the fingertips, may be an early change. Posterior column and pyramidal tract involvement result in more severe abnormalities— unsteadiness of gait, weakness of the lower limbs and paralysis of the bladder. Early in the involvement of the nervous system, vibration sense at the malleoli is always impaired. Toe position and tendo Achillis sensation are usually reduced. The Romberg sign is commonly positive. A spastic paraplegia completes the picture of severe spinal cord involvement. Evidence of intellectual impairment, sometimes of a severe degree, and even a florid psychosis may be found in patients long untreated.

(e) *Minerals*

(i) *Iron deficiency anaemia*

Patients suffering from this common condition are rarely psychotic. It is doubtful whether one should classify iron deficiency as a cause of psychosis. On rare occasions it is a contributing factor; the correction of the anaemia brings about improvement in the mental state. The main features are: a hypochromic, microcytic anaemia, with spooned nails and a smooth tongue if the anaemia has been persistently severe. In men and post-menopausal women, gastro-intestinal bleeding due to ulceration is much the most frequent cause.

(ii) *Calcium deficiency* (hypocalcaemia)

Only rarely would one encounter this condition in psychiatric practice. None the less, psychosis, mental deficiency and epilepsy occur in some patients suffering from hypocalcaemia. Tetany is the most common presenting manifestation.

The causes can be divided into three groups. First, there may be a dietary deficiency of calcium or vitamin D resulting in rickets in children and osteomalacia in adults. Secondly, extensive bowel disease or surgical resection of bowel may cause steatorrhoea, with secondary calcium deficiency resulting from poor intestinal absorption. Thirdly, hypoparathyroidism can be responsible. Nearly always the cause of hypoparathyroidism is accidental removal of the parathyroid glands during a thyroidectomy. (It is wise to make a careful appraisal of parathyroid and thyroid function in any mentally ill patient who has had a thyroidectomy.) Those cases of hypoparathyroidism of unknown cause are listed as idiopathic. If hypoparathyroidism is unrecognized for a long time, profound mental changes may take place. Onset of the disease in childhood may result in mental deficiency. Frequently, patients with hypoparathyroidism have epileptic seizures; attacks of tetany are commonly observed, but tetany may remain either latent or a minor feature of the disease. If cerebral calcification (usually most marked in the basal ganglia) can be demonstrated, the diagnosis becomes clear. Deposition of calcium in the lens produces cataracts which may seriously impair vision. Serum calcium levels are low in contrast with the high concentrations of serum phosphorus.

(iii) *Calcium excess* (hypercalcaemia)

Usually this is due to hyperparathyroidism. Such patients, because they are often weak, irritable and bothered by vaguely localized pain due to the bone changes, may be erroneously considered to have a neurosis. Very occasionally, the patient may be psychotic.

Clinically there may be one or more of the following features: Increased thirst and polyuria can occur as a direct result of the high level of blood calcium, which brings about an increased excretion of calcium in the urine causing a diuresis. Kidney stones may cause renal or ureteral colic, haematuria or renal infections. Spontaneous fracture may be the first clinical feature to direct attention to osteitis fibrosa cystica. The parathyroid tumour, though usually small, may be sufficiently large to be palpable in the region of the thyroid gland.

Laboratory tests will show elevation of the serum calcium and depression of the serum phosphorus levels. In the presence of bone changes, the alkaline phosphatase content of serum will be increased.

(iv) *Disordered copper metabolism*

Hepato-lenticular degeneration or Wilson's disease is a rare, frequently familial condition, in which there is dysfunction of the basal ganglia giving rise to tremor and rigidity, accompanied by cirrhosis of the liver. The onset is usually in adolescence with a tremor which is characteristically flapping, rigidity, mask-like facies, inappropriate emotional outbursts and mental deterioration. A greenish-brown ring of copper is deposited around the cornea. There is retention of copper salts in the brain and liver. British Anti-Lewisite (BAL), which induces an increased excretion of copper in the urine, has been found useful in therapy.

(f) *Porphyrins*

Porphyria

This is a rare disease and because of its many different manifestations probably often overlooked. Symptoms and signs are widespread, a fact which is not surprising since porphyrins are involved in the basic metabolic processes of all cells. The adult form may occur sporadically or in several members of the same family. Some drugs, particularly barbiturates and sulphonal compounds, may precipitate attacks. Females are affected more often than males. Patients often have a photosensitive skin with a rash on exposed areas. Abdominal pain of various types and locations occurs in bouts and may result in fruitless surgery. Hypertension and retinopathy are sometimes found. Neurotic and psychotic mental states of almost all types may be prominent. Peripheral neuropathy with predominantly motor abnormalities, particularly marked muscle wasting, has often been seen. The urine is intermittently wine-coloured, especially if exposed to sunlight. Porphobilinogen should be sought for by using the Ehrlich reagent but repeated tests may be necessary because the excretion of porphobilinogen varies from day to day. (See Technical Procedures p. 161).

(g) *Electrolytes*

(See section (*j*) on hormones for a description of well-marked electrolyte disturbances occurring in association with psychoses as a result of altered adrenal function. Other conditions which give rise to excessive vomiting or diarrhoea may produce severe electrolyte upsets.)

(h) *Acid Base Balance* (pH)

Disturbances in acid base balance do not occur as isolated events but are found in association with alterations of the equilibrium of fluids and electrolytes. A good example is the severe alkalosis which develops in some patients with Cushing's syndrome who have elevation of serum sodium together with decrease in serum potassium and chloride. Delirium may appear under such circumstances and then clear up completely when the alkalosis and electrolyte abnormalities are corrected.

(i) *Water*

Dehydration may, in some instances, be a contributing or

aggravating factor in a psychosis. It should be emphasized, however, that the body is remarkably efficient in its adaptation to dehydration and cerebral function is usually not grossly impaired.

(j) Hormones
(i) Pituitary
Anterior pituitary insufficiency. Psychiatrists should be familiar with this disease not only because psychosis is sometimes a feature but also because anterior pituitary insufficiency bears a superficial resemblance to anorexia nervosa.

The cause is decreased functioning of anterior pituitary tissue. Most of the patients are women who have had severe post-partum haemorrhage, shock, and presumably infarction of the anterior portion of the pituitary. Lactation may never commence or may cease prematurely. In the ensuing months there may be loss of libido, loss of axillary and pubic hair, atrophy of the genitalia, features of adrenal insufficiency and thyroid insufficiency, which are described in the following two sections. Thus, the clinical syndrome of anterior pituitary insufficiency is the result of a deficiency in the production of the trophic hormones, namely the thyrotrophic, adrenocorticotrophic, gonadotrophic, and lactogenic hormones. Theoretically, any extensive lesion of the anterior pituitary could be responsible. Gumma, tuberculoma, tumour or atrophy of unknown cause have been described.

(ii) Adrenal
Adrenal cortical insufficiency (Addison's disease). The psychiatric manifestations of this disease are becoming more widely recognized. Patients may be anxious, depressed, retarded, schizoid or floridly paranoidal.

There are many other clinical findings in Addison's disease. Gastrointestinal symptoms include anorexia, weight loss, nausea, vomiting and diarrhoea. There is brown or bluish-black pigmentation of the buccal mucosa, exposed skin and pressure points where skin overlies bone as in the scapular areas. Infection may play one of two parts: tuberculosis of the adrenal glands, no longer the commonest cause of adrenal insufficiency for it now ranks after adrenal atrophy, may be present in association with tuberculous infection elsewhere; during infections of various kinds, adrenal insufficiency may become profound. Crises resulting from hypoglycaemia and severe electrolyte disturbance with sodium chloride deficit give rise to a state of shock. Hypotension, present throughout the disease, is more marked during crises.

Abnormal blood chemistry findings consist of hypoglycaemia with a flat glucose tolerance curve, low concentrations of serum sodium and chloride, and a high concentration of serum potassium. The number of lymphocytes and eosinophiles in the blood is increased .

Adrenal cortical hyperfunction (Cushing's syndrome). This is due to an excess of adrenal cortical hormones. Therapy with the adrenocorticotrophic hormone and cortisone, as well as adrenal cortical tumour or hyperplasia are the common causes. It is debatable whether tumour or hyperplasia of the anterior lobe of the pituitary gland may produce Cushing's syndrome.

Adrenocorticotrophic hormone (ACTH) and cortisone have the effect on some people of producing a striking euphoria with increased appetite and sense of well-being. In a few, severe psychosis results. Psychosis is also a feature in a considerable number of cases of Cushing's syndrome due to adrenal cortical disease.

The chief characteristics of Cushing's syndrome are as follows: The altered distribution of body fat, coupled with the steady protein loss, produces a round-faced, thick-necked individual with an obese trunk often capped by fat pads on the shoulders. In contrast, the arms and legs decrease in bulk. Patients usually complain of marked muscular weakness. Hirsutism, more readily noticeable in women, may attract attention. The skin becomes thin, bruises easily, and particularly over the thighs and abdomen purplish striae appear.

Nearly all patients have hypertension. Some become diabetic, the blood sugar sometimes being difficult to control with insulin. Osteoporosis, another evidence of protein loss, commonly results in kyphosis. Polycythaemia sometimes occurs. Eosinopoenia is an important feature for, unless there be some coincidental cause for eosinophilia such as an allergic condition, the eosinophil count will usually be less than 50 per c. mm. The excretion of adrenal steroids in the urine is increased: about half the patients excrete excessive quantities of 17-ketosteroids and nearly all patients excrete more glucocorticoids than normal persons. In some cases in which the illness runs a rather acute course, the level of serum potassium may be low and be associated with severe alkalosis.

(iii) *Thyroid*

Hyperthyroidism. There is a close similarity between some patients with hyperthyroidism and patients who have anxiety states. The differentiation is most important because hyperthyroidism sometimes has a fatal outcome if unrecognized. The thyrotoxic patient may be restless, tremulous, agitated and anxious, or maniacal and delirious.

The main features of thyrotoxicosis can be divided into several groups. The hypermetabolism results in a warm, moist skin, and accelerated cardiac action in the form of sinus tachycardia or auricular fibrillation which may lead to cardiac failure. Usually there is restlessness, a fine rapid finger tremor, increased appetite, loss of weight, weakness, heat intolerance and occasionally myopathy in the form of focal muscle wasting or myasthenia gravis. A goitre is almost always detectable, though it may be hidden behind the sternum; often a bruit is audible over the goitre. Exophthalmos is frequently present. If the output of thyroid hormone from a hyperfunctioning thyroid gland is rapid and excessive, thyroid storm may result. In this condition the patient is very restless, feverish, dehydrated and may become maniacal. The symptoms and signs of hyperthyroidism are present to an unusually severe degree.

There are three valuable laboratory procedures: determinations of the basal metabolic rate, the concentration of protein-bound iodine in the serum and the measurement of the uptake of radioactive iodine by the thyroid gland. In hyperthyroidism these three tests give higher results than normal.

Hypothyroidism (myxoedema). Mental functions are usually slowed down but emotional responses, though flat, are not qualitatively altered. There is commonly impairment of memory and inability to perform rapid calculations. In a few patients, thinking, mood and behaviour are definitely psychotic, with paranoid trends being a common feature.

The skin becomes coarse, thick, dry, and, especially around the eyes, puffy. The hair also coarsens, loses its slightly moist quality and becomes sparse, particularly at the outer third of the eyebrows. The voice is hoarse and croaking. Deafness is common. The patient notices an intolerance of cold. Enlargement of the cardiac outline, with or without heart failure, often occurs and the electrocardiogram reveals bradycardia, low voltage and flattened T-waves.

The laboratory tests mentioned under hyperthyroidism show subnormal values. Frequently the amount of protein in the cerebrospinal fluid is increased above normal values.

(k) Oxygen

As has been stated, the nerve cell is very sensitive to deprivation of oxygen. Clinically, there are two main patterns of mental disturbance depending on the severity and duration of the oxygen lack. Where the brain is inadequately supplied with oxygen for minutes or a few hours, and where the degree of anoxaemia is not profound, transient delirium may occur. But if there be prolonged, more profound, oxygen lack, cerebral damage will be severe and the outcome is chronic dementia.

Theoretically, the clinical setting might be that associated with any cause of cerebral cell anoxia. These are listed briefly in section 1, sub-section (k), of the aetiological classification.

Actually, there are only a few important conditions met in practice.

Even in cardiac or pulmonary failure of disabling degree, the gasping, cyanosed patient is usually quite free of grossly disordered thinking or disturbance of mood. A few elderly patients with cardiac failure and associated cerebral athero-sclerosis have paranoid, confused, delirious periods, often only at night, which disappear when the cardiac failure is success-fully treated. The diagnostic features of cardiac and respiratory disease severe enough to cause cerebral anoxia are so obvious that they require no comment.

Severe anaemia, resulting in anoxaemia, has already been discussed under Vitamin B_{12} and iron deficiency.

Carbon monoxide poisoning, a not uncommon condition, results from occupational, accidental, suicidal or homicidal exposure. Usually the source of the gas is exhaust from an automobile engine. The danger of exposure to carbon mon-oxide gas lies in the fact that haemoglobin has a much stronger affinity for carbon monoxide than for oxygen, with the result that much of the haemoglobin is no longer available for trans-porting oxygen. If the patient is exposed to high concentrations of carbon monoxide, there is a rapid, painless onset of coma. A period of headache, dizziness and nausea may precede the coma if exposure is to smaller concentrations. At this stage the blood has a bright, cherry-red colour which tints the muco-sal surfaces. If the blood is examined spectroscopically within a few hours of exposure, it is possible to demonstrate carboxy-haemoglobin. The outcome is dependent on the severity of exposure. There may be either complete recovery, a lingering period of emotional lability and slight intellectual deteriora-tion, or varying degrees of dementia. During the ensuing months, Parkinsonism may accompany evidence of organic mental changes. In some cases air studies have shown diffuse enlargement of the ventricular system.

The most dramatic setting for cerebral anoxia is cardiac arrest. Many instances have been recorded during operations under general anaesthesia. The cerebral cortex deprived of oxygen for a period exceeding approximately ten minutes will be irreversibly damaged, the frontal cortex being most sensitive to the deprivation.

Regardless of the cause of the cerebral anoxia, the result depends upon the severity and duration of the anoxia, the mental sequelae ranging from little or no intellectual deterioration to a decerebrate state. In some cases improvement may take place and this may be facilitated by a skilful programme of rehabilitation.

Undoubtedly many drugs interfere with intracellular oxidation reactions. The exact enzymatic derangements are poorly understood in most cases, although cyanide and carbon monoxide, for example, are known to inhibit cytochrome oxidase.

REFERENCES

(a) *Carbohydrate*

BLACK, K. O., CORBETT, R. S., HOSFORD, J. P. and TURNER, J. W. A.: Spontaneous hyperinsulinism due to islet-cell adenoma, Brit.M.J. 1:55, Jan. 9, 1954.

BREIDAHL, H. D., PRIESTLEY, J. T. and RYNEARSON, E. H.: Hyperinsulinism: Surgical aspects and results, Ann. Surg. 142:698, Oct. 1955.

BROWN, H., HARGREAVES, H. P. and TYLER, F. H.: Islet-cell adenoma of the pancreas, Arch. Int. Med. 89:951, June 1952.

CONN, J. W. and SELTZER, H. S.: Spontaneous hypoglycaemia, Am. J. Med. 19:460, Sept. 1955.

FINEBERG, S. K. and ALTSCHUL, A.: The encephalopathy of hyperinsulinism, Ann. Int. Med. 36:536, Feb. 1952.

LIEBERMAN, A. A.: Nervous and mental manifestations observed in spontaneous hypoglycaemia, Elgin Papers 5:43, Dec. 1944.

MORLEY, J.: Insulin tumours of the pancreas, Brit. J. Surg. 40:97, Sept. 1952.

RICHARDSON, J. E. and RUSSELL, D. S.: Cerebral disease due to functioning islet-cell tumours, Lancet 263:1054, Nov. 29, 1952.

SMITH, A. N. and COCHRAN, J. B.: Islet-cell tumour of the pancreas, Lancet 262:289, Feb. 9, 1952.

WELLS, J. S.: Case of hypoglycaemia committed to a mental hospital, Psychiat. Quart. 17:672, Oct. 1943.

(b) *Fat*

BRAIN, W. R.: Diseases of the Nervous System, ed. 5, Toronto, Oxford Medical Publications, 1955, pp. 584–589.

LOKEN, A. C. and CYVIN, K.: A case of clinical juvenile amaurotic idiocy with the histological picture of Alzheimer's disease, J. Neurol. Neurosurg. & Psychiat. 17:211, Aug. 1954.

(c) *Protein and Amino Acids*

ALVORD, E. C., JR., STEVENSON, L. D., VOGEL, F. S. and ENGLE, R. L., JR.: Neuropathological findings in phenylpyruvic oligophrenia (phenylketonuria), J. Neuropath. & Exper. Neurol. 9:298, July 1950.

CAWTE, J. E.: Phenylketonuria, M. J. Australia 41:15, July 3, 1954.

EDITORIAL: Phenylpyruvic oligophrenia, Ann. Int. Med. 44:819, April 1956.

FOIS, A., ROSENBERG, C. and GIBBS, F. A.: The electroencephalogram in phenylpyruvic oligophrenia, Electroencephalog. & Clin. Neurophysiol. 7:569, Nov. 1955.

HORNER, F. A. and STREAMER, C. W.: Effect of a phenylalanine-restricted diet on patients with phenylketonuria, J.A.M.A. 161:1628, Aug. 25, 1956.

JERVIS, G. A.: Phenylpyruvic oligophrenia, Arch. Neurol. & Psychiat. 38:944, Nov. 1937.

JOSEPHY, H.: Phenylpyruvic oligophrenia, Illinois M.J. 94:107, Aug. 1948.

PENROSE, L. S.: Inheritance of phenylpyruvic amentia (phenylketonuria), Lancet 228:192, July 27, 1935.

(d) *Vitamin Deficiencies*

ASSOCIATION FOR RESEARCH IN NERVOUS AND MENTAL DISEASE: Vol. XXII, The Role of Nutritional Deficiency in Nervous and Mental Diseases, Baltimore, Williams and Wilkins Co., 1943.

SPILLANE, J. D.: Nutritional Disorders of the Nervous System, Edinburgh, E. & S. Livingstone Ltd., 1947.

(i) *Thiamine deficiency*

DENNY-BROWN, D. and FOLEY, J. M.: Clinical pathologic conference, Neurology 5:510, July 1955.

JOLLIFFE, N., WORTIS, H. and FEIN, H. D.: The Wernicke syndrome, Arch. Neurol. & Psychiat. 46:569, Oct. 1941.

MALAMUD, N. and SKILLICORN, S. A.: Relationship between the Wernicke and Korsakoff syndrome, Arch. Neurol. & Psychiat. 76:585, Dec. 1956.

VICTOR, M. and YAKOVLEV, P. I.: S. S. Korsakoff's psychic disorder in conjunction with peripheral neuritis: A translation of Korsakoff's original article with brief comments on the author and his contribution to clinical medicine, Neurology 5:394, June 1955.

(ii) *Nicotinic acid deficiency*

ALESHIRE, I: Delusion of parasitosis, J.A.M.A. 155:15, May 1, 1954.

DEWAN, J. G.: The etiology of pellagra, Am. J. Psychiat. 97:1188, March 1941.

GREGORY, I.: The role of nicotinic acid (niacin) in mental health and disease, J. Ment. Sc. 101:85, Jan. 1955.

HERSOV, L. A.: A case of childhood pellagra with psychosis, J. Ment. Sc. 101:878, Oct. 1955.

MEYERSBURG, H. A.: Senile psychosis and pellagra, New England J. Med. 233:173, Aug. 9, 1945.

RODNIGHT, R. and McILWAIN, H.: Indicanuria and the psychosis of a pellagrin, J. Ment. Sc. 101:884, Oct. 1955.

SPIES, T. D. (Guest Editor): Pellagrous psychosis, Postgrad. Med. 17:70, March 1955.

(iii) *Vitamin B₁₂ deficiency*

HOLMES, J. M.: Cerebral manifestations of vitamin B_{12} deficiency, Brit. M.J. 2:1394, Dec. 15, 1956.

SAMSON, D. C., SWISHER, S. M., CHRISTIAN, R. M. and ENGEL, G. L.: Cerebral metabolic disturbance and delirium in pernicious anaemia: Clinical and electroencephalographic studies, Arch. Int. Med. 90:4, July 1952.

WALTON, J. N., KILOH, L. G., OSSELTON, J. W. and FARRALL, J.: The electroencephalogram in pernicious anaemia and subacute combined degeneration of the cord, Electroencephalog. & Clin. Neurophysiol. 6:45, Feb. 1954.

(e) *Minerals*
    (ii) *Calcium deficiency*

BAILEY, D. S. G. M., DONOVAN, J. F. and GALBRAITH, A. J.: Clinical and EEG aspects of psychiatric disorders associated with tetany, J. Ment. Sc. 98:618, Oct. 1952.

KAYE, M., STACEY, C. H. and ROSENFELD, I.: Psychosis following removal of a parathyroid adenoma for hyperparathyroidism, Canad. M.A.J. 72:214, Feb. 1, 1955.

ROBINSON, K. C., KALLBERG, M. H. and CROWLEY, M. F.: Idiopathic hypoparathyroidism presenting as dementia, Brit. M.J. 2:1203, Nov. 20, 1954.

SCARLETT, E. P. and HOUGHTLING, W. J.: Psychosis in hypoparathyroidism, Canad. M.A.J. 50:351, April 1944.

SIMPSON, J. A.: The neurological manifestations of idiopathic hypoparathyroidism, Brain 75:76, 1952.

SUGAR, O.: Central neurological complications of hypoparathyroidism, Arch. Neurol. & Psychiat. 70:86, July 1953.

(iii) *Calcium excess*

FITZ, T. E. and HALLMAN, B. L.: Mental changes associated with hyperparathyroidism, Arch. Int. Med. 89:547, April 1952.

NIELSEN, H.: Familial occurrence, gastrointestinal symptoms and mental disturbances in hyperparathyroidism, Acta med. scandinav. 151:359, 1955.

(iv) *Disordered copper metabolism*

BRENNER, C., FRIEDMAN, A. P. and MERRITT, H. H.: Psychiatric syndromes in patients with organic brain disease, I, Diseases of the basal ganglia, Am. J. Psychiat. 103:733, May 1947.

EDITORIAL: Hepato-lenticular degeneration, Brit. M.J. 1:218, Jan. 28, 1956.

(v) *Others*

FLINK, E. B.: Magnesium deficiency syndrome in man, J.A.M.A. 160:1406, April 21, 1956.

FLINK, E. B., STUTZMAN, F. L., ANDERSON, A. R., KONIG, T. and FRASER, R.: Magnesium deficiency after prolonged parenteral fluid administration and after chronic alcoholism complicated by delirium tremens, J. Lab. and Clin. Med. 43:169, Feb. 1954.

SUTER, C. and KLINGMAN, W. O.: Neurologic manifestations of magnesium depletion states, Neurology 5:691, Oct. 1955.

(*f*) *Porphyrins*

HIRSH, S. and DUNSWORTH, F. A.: An interesting case of porphyria, Am. J. Psychiat. 111:703, March 1955.

MARKOVITZ, M.: Acute intermittent porphyria: A report of five cases and a review of the literature, Ann. Int. Med. 41:1170, Dec. 1954.

PETERS, H. A., WOODS, S., EICHMAN, P. L. and REESE, H. H.: The treatment of acute porphyria with chelating agents: A report of 21 cases, Ann. Int. Med. 47:889, Nov. 1957.

ROTH, N.: The neuropsychiatric aspects of porphyria, Psychosom. Med. 7:291, Sept. 1945.

(*g*) *Electrolytes*

SPAULDING, W. B., OILLE, W. A. and GORNALL, A. G.: Mineralocorticoid-like disturbance associated with adrenal metastases from a bronchogenic carcinoma, Ann. Int. Med. 42:444, Feb. 1955. (Case 5, chap. XII.)

WELTI, W.: Delirium with low serum sodium, Arch. Neurol. & Psychiat. 76:559, Nov. 1956.

(*j*) *Hormones*

(i) *Pituitary—anterior pituitary insufficiency*

CRAIG, L. S.: Simulated endocrine disorders, Am. Pract. & Digest Treat. 3:957, Dec. 1952.

FARQUHARSON, F. R.: Simmonds' Disease, Springfield, Ill., C. C. Thomas, 1950.

SEXTON, D. L., MORTON, R. F. and SAXTON, J.: Simmonds' disease, J. Clin. Endocrinol. 10:1417, Nov. 1950.

TODD, J.: A case of Simmonds's disease with mental symptoms, Brit. M.J. 2:569, Sept. 8, 1951.

(ii) *Adrenal—adrenal cortical insufficiency*
CLEGHORN, R. A.: Adrenal cortical insufficiency: psychological and neurological observations, Canad. M.A.J. 65:449, Nov. 1951.

GORMAN, W. F. and WORTIS, S. B.: Psychosis in Addison's disease, Dis. Nerv. System 8:267, Sept. 1947.

Adrenal cortical hyperfunction
ABBOTT, W. E., JEFFRIES, W. McK., LEVEY, S. and KRIEGER, H.: Total bilateral adrenalectomy for adrenal cortical hyperfunction, J.A.M.A. 156:1168, Nov. 20, 1954.

HAMM, F. C.: Adrenal surgery for psychoses associated with Cushing's syndrome, Arch. Surg. 71:617, Oct. 1955.

HERTZ, P. E., NADAS, E. and WOJTKOWSKI, H.: Cushings's syndrome and its management, Am. J. Psychiat. 112:144, Aug. 1955.

MACLAY, W. S., and STOKES, A. B.: Mental disorder in Cushing's syndrome, J. Neurol. & Psychiat. 1:110, April 1938.

SPILLANE, J. D.: Nervous and mental disorders in Cushing's syndrome, Brain 74:72, Part I, 1951.

STARR, A. M.: Personality changes in Cushing's syndrome, J. Clin. Endocrinol. 12:502, May 1952.

TRETHOWAN, W. H. and COBB, S.: Neuropsychiatric aspects of Cushing's syndrome, Arch. Neurol. & Psychiat. 67:283, March 1952.

(iii) *Thyroid—Hyperthyroidism*
HENDERSON, D. K. and GILLESPIE, R. D.: A Textbook of Psychiatry, ed. 8, Toronto, Oxford University Press, 1956, pp. 536–539.

MEANS, J. H.: The Thyroid and its Diseases, ed. 2, Montreal, J. B. Lippincott Co., 1948, pp. 276–278, 430–432.

THOMPSON, G. N.: Self-induced psychosis with hyperthyroidism complicating manic depressive psychosis, Am. J. Psychiat. 102:395, Nov. 1945.

Hypothyroidism
ASHER, R.: Myxoedematous madness, Brit. M.J. 2:555, Sept. 10, 1949.

CALVERT, R. J., SMITH, E. and ANDREWS, L. G.: Coexistent myxoedema heart disease and psychosis, Brit. M.J. 2:891, Oct. 16, 1954.

CHAMBERS, W. N. and MILNE, J.: Myxedema in two brothers, one with psychosis, Ann. Int. Med. 43:892, Oct. 1955.

REITAN, R. M.: Intellectual functions in myxedema, Arch. Neurol. & Psychiat. 69:436, April 1953.

(k) *Oxygen*
BEDFORD, P. D.: Adverse cerebral effects of anaesthesia on old people, Lancet 269:259, Aug. 6, 1955.

FREEMAN, R. V., BERGER, L. M., COHEN, S. and SELLE, W. A.: Major neuropsychiatric. residuals following resuscitation from cardiac arrest, J.A.M.A. 155:107, May 8, 1954.

TURNER, H.: Case report: The mental state during recovery after heart arrest during anaesthesia, J. Neurol. Neurosurg. & Psychiat. 13:153, May 1950.

CHAPTER IV

Disordered Blood Supply of Cerebral Cells

(a) Cerebral Atherosclerosis

The most common vascular disease impairing cerebral circulation is atherosclerosis. However, in any given patient it is difficult to be sure that atherosclerosis of cerebral arteries is definitely present. One seeks evidence of atherosclerosis elsewhere in the body, always remembering that the arterial change may be much more extensive in one part of the vascular bed than another. For example, the coronary arteries may be severely affected, resulting in angina pectoris and myocardial infarction while, at the same time, cerebral arteries are much less involved and cerebral function unimpaired. Long-standing hypertension and diabetes accelerate atherosclerosis and, therefore, provide a commonly encountered clinical background for the condition. Thickening of superficial arteries such as the brachial, radial or temporal (Mönckeberg's medial degeneration) is quite different from atherosclerosis and no clinical inference regarding cerebral circulation should be drawn from its presence.

When considering psychosis due to cerebral atherosclerosis, several factors should be kept in mind. The adequacy of cerebral circulation varies from time to time. A fall in blood pressure due to any cause will impair the supply of blood to the brain; slowing of circulation due to cardiac insufficiency, even in the presence of a normally maintained blood pressure, may have the same effect. Cerebral vascular spasm is a much disputed mechanism of cerebral ischaemia. Certainly some hypertensive patients experience sudden, brief episodes with such symptoms as severe headache, dizziness, fainting, mental confusion, paraesthesias and pareses, but whether spasm underlies is not definitely known. Recently there has been considerable attention paid to occlusion of the common or internal carotid arteries by thrombus: such an occurrence may leave the cerebral circulation in a precarious state, such that hypotension or slowing of circulation could cause transient cerebral dysfunction. Careful clinico-pathological studies have failed to reveal any consistently positive correlation between the severity of mental deterioration and the degree of cerebral atherosclerosis. Psychological factors probably play a major part in determining the appearance of mental symptoms.

It is commonly taught that one requisite for the diagnosis of psychosis due to cerebral atherosclerosis is clinical evidence of focal brain damage. A transient stroke or Jacksonian seizures may have occurred. We feel, however, that in persons in their fifties or sixties, with the onset of organic mental symptoms such as failing memory, emotional lability, impaired judgment and intellectual efficiency but no other evidence of any other form of cerebral disease, a provisional diagnosis of psychosis due to cerebral atherosclerosis may be made. There are exacerbations and remissions of the symptoms, rather than a steady course of progressive deterioration. In such cases the diagnosis of cerebral arteriosclerosis is probably correct but impossible to prove with certainty, even at autopsy.

(b) Thrombosis

Commonly, cerebral function is impaired by the infarction of a large area of brain tissue or by multiple infarctions of small areas. It is rare, however, for such a patient to be floridly psychotic. Usually, the history is one of initial maximal disability of the nervous system followed by gradual improvement. Indications of localized brain damage are often found, for example, aphasia, paresis or hemianopia. Of the various vascular diseases which predispose to arterial thrombosis, atherosclerosis is much the most common.

Syphilis of the meningovascular type is characterized by an endarteritis which may lead to thrombosis and cerebral infarction. In such a setting psychosis would be unusual unless the parenchymal cerebral changes of general paresis coexisted. Pure meningovascular syphilis usually appears a few years after the primary infection and often manifests itself by signs of a meningitis or by cranial nerve abnormalities, such as diplopia due to ocular muscle palsy. The cerebrospinal fluid shows a positive Wasserman test, increase in lymphocytes, elevated protein content and sometimes a mid-zone rise in the colloidal gold curve.

Cortical venous thrombosis is not as rare as has been thought. It occurs in the same setting as venous thrombosis in the legs: after operations and childbirth, in cardiac failure and in cachectic states. Psychosis is a rare manifestation. Cortical sensory loss of vision, two-point discrimination and stereognosis may occur, as well as cortical motor loss in the form of paresis usually confined to half the body.

(c) *Haemorrhage*

Cerebral haemorrhage is a common occurrence which often produces death but rarely a psychosis. Usually the vessels are diseased and often the presence of hypertension contributes to the rupture of vessel wall. Hypertension often accompanies atherosclerosis and always accompanies arteriolosclerosis or, the more malignant stage, arteriolonecrosis.

Subarachnoid haemorrhage is usually due to rupture of a congenital "berry" aneurysm. Patients with this condition are younger, on the average, than those in whom haemorrhage occurs upon rupture of degenerated vessels. The extracranial arteries may be quite normal. Sudden, severe occipital headache with drowsiness often progressing to coma are the outstanding features. The spinal fluid is grossly bloody. Mental impairment sometimes occurs as a sequel to subarachnoid haemorrhage.

(d) Embolism

Psychosis only rarely is brought about by embolism with subsequent infarction. In addition to recognizing the disorder of the central nervous system, a site of origin for the embolus must be demonstrated to make this diagnosis. Commonly emboli arise from the thrombi which have formed either on diseased heart valves as, for example, in subacute bacterial endocarditis, or on the endocardial surface of infarcted heart walls or in the appendages of dilated auricles contracting poorly because of auricular fibrillation. After fractures, showers of fat emboli may be carried to the brain producing both acute psychosis and chronic dementia. The finding of droplets of fat in sputum or urine confirms the diagnosis.

(e) Slowing of Blood Flow

Elderly patients, commonly with cerebral atherosclerosis, may become confused or delirious if they develop cardiac failure. The mental disturbance which is often worse at night may clear in a few hours or days.

(f) Less Common Types of Vascular Disease

Polyarteritis nodosa, though uncommon, deserves consideration because psychotic episodes may be part of the clinical picture. This diffuse vascular disease usually affects males in early adult life. The clinical manifestations are most variegated because any small artery can be involved. Asthma, hypertension, peripheral neuritis, myocardial infarction and pulmonary infarction are some of the possible results. Fever, leucocytosis, eosinophilia, and signs of renal disease, especially albuminuria and haematuria, may be found. Sometimes a biopsy of skin and muscle reveals the diagnostic microscopic changes in the small arteries.

Another form of diffuse collagen disease, *systemic lupus erythematosus*, may cause organic psychosis. Systemic lupus erythematosus is a disease of connective tissue which usually affects young women. The manifestations, like those of polyarteritis nodosa, are protean because the lesions may occur anywhere in the body. The skin is commonly affected and areas exposed to sunlight become erythematous, dry and scaly, the most characteristic lesion being a rash over the bridge of the nose extending over the cheeks. Serous membranes may be involved with pleurisy, pericarditis and peritonitis being common examples. Synovial membranes react in a manner sometimes indistinguishable from the changes of rheumatoid arthritis. The walls of small arteries and capillaries are commonly affected, endocarditis may occur and renal damage frequently gives rise to albuminuria, abnormalities of the urinary sediment and later uraemia. Often there are one or more abnormalities of the blood such as haemolytic anaemia, leucopoenia or thrombocytopoenia commonly with splenomegaly. Neurological manifestations include epileptic fits, cranial and peripheral nerve abnormalities and mental disturbances of a confusional type. The hypersensitivity to drugs so often found, coupled with the photosensitivity of the skin and the types of haematological disturbance, suggests that the disease may prove to be an "auto-immune" disorder in which the patient develops antibodies against his own cells. The diagnosis of this serious disease is much facilitated by the "L-E cell" test which is positive at some time or other in the course of the disease in most patients.

Temporal arteritis is a disease of older people in which granulomatous changes occur in the walls of certain arteries. Cranial vessels, particularly the temporals, are most affected, but sometimes arteries elsewhere in the body take part in the process. The commonest symptom is severe headache, accompanied by tenderness over the diseased artery, fever, leucocytosis and increased sedimentation rate. General symptoms of weakness, weight loss and anorexia are prominent. Blindness may result from impairment of the blood supply to the eyes. A few patients have been described in whom confusion, delirium or depression were outstanding findings.

REFERENCES

ALLEN, E. B.: Psychiatric aspects of cerebral arteriosclerosis, New England J. Med. 245:677, Nov. 1, 1951.

ALPERS, B. J., FORSTER, F. M. and HERBUT, P. A.: Retinal, cerebral and systemic arteriosclerosis, Arch. Neurol. & Psychiat. 60:440, Nov. 1948.

BEDFORD, P. D.: Adverse cerebral effects following acute haemorrhage in elderly people, Lancet 271:750, Oct. 13, 1956.

CLARK, E. and HARRISON, C. V.: Bilateral carotid artery obstruction, Neurology 6:705, Oct. 1956.

CLARK, E. C. and BAILEY, A. A.: Neurological and psychiatric signs associated with systemic lupus erythematosus, J.A.M.A. 160:455, Feb. 11, 1956.

FISHER, M.: Occlusion of the carotid arteries, Arch. Neurol. & Psychiat. 72:187, Aug. 1954.

FRENCH, L. A. and PEYTON, W. T.: Vascular malformations in the region of the great vein of Galen, J. Neurosurg. 11:488, Sept. 1954.

GLASER, G. H.: Lesions of the central nervous system in disseminated lupus erythematosus, Arch. Neurol. & Psychiat. 67:745, June 1952.

HUGHES, W., DODGSON, M. C. H. and MacLENNAN, D. C.: Chronic cerebral hypertensive disease, Lancet 267:770, Oct. 16, 1954.

MacKAY, M. E., McLARDY, T. and HARRIS, C.: A case of periarteritis nodosa of the central nervous system, J. Ment. Sc. 96:470, April 1950.

ROTHSCHILD, D.: Neuropathologic changes in arteriosclerotic psychoses and their psychiatric significance, Arch. Neurol. & Psychiat. 48:417, Sept. 1942.

SEDGWICK, R. P. and VON HAGEN, K. O.: The neurological manifestation of lupus erythematosus and periarteritis nodosa, Bull. Los Angeles Neurol. Soc. 13:129, Sept. 1948.

SHAPIRO, S. K. and PEYTON, W. T.: Spontaneous thrombosis of the carotid arteries, Neurology 4:83, Feb. 1954.

STEVENS, H.: Puerperal hemiplegia, Neurology 4:723, Oct. 1954.

VEREKER, R.: The psychiatric aspects of temporal arteritis, J. Ment. Sc. 98:280, April 1952.

WALTON, J. N.: The late prognosis of subarachnoid haemorrhage, Brit. M.J. 2:802, Oct. 11, 1952.

CHAPTER V

Mechanical Stresses Interfering with Cerebral Cell Function

(a) *Space-Occupying Lesions*

Such lesions produce effects which may be grouped as follows:

(i) those due to the pathological nature of the lesion;
(ii) those due to increased intracranial pressure;
(iii) those dependent on the particular location of the lesion in the brain.

Brain tumours may be primary or secondary. Because primary brain tumours almost never metastasize outside the skull, their clinical effects are due to increased intracranial pressure and localized dysfunction or a combination of the two. Headache is a common symptom regardless of whether the intracranial pressure be elevated or not. Raised intracranial pressure gives rises to vomiting, impairment of consciousness and papilloedema. Under these latter circumstances, lumbar puncture is contra-indicated because of the danger of oedematous hippocampal unci herniating through the tentorium cerebelli or the cerebellar tonsils herniating through the foramen magnum thereby producing compression of the brain stem. Brain tumours give rise to manifold localizing neurological phenomena including focal fits of sensory or motor type, visual disturbances such as hemionopia, paralyses and sensory abnormalities. The mental symptoms that are frequently associated with brain tumour may vary from a functional picture to delirium, dementia or coma. In approximately half the cases of secondary brain tumours there are associated neoplastic deposits in the lungs, because bronchogenic carcinoma commonly metastasizes to brain and because primary malignant tumours of other organs, for example, the bowel or kidney, commonly metastasize to lungs as well as to brain. The chest should be X-rayed in every patient suspected of having a brain tumour.

Haemorrhage may act as a space-occupying lesion. The commonest condition behaving in this manner is subdural haematoma. Usually a history of head injury, often trivial, and occurring days, weeks, or even months before the onset of symptoms may be elicited. The patient is commonly middle-aged or elderly, often alcoholic, sometimes chronically psychotic. Alcoholism and disturbed behaviour of course carry a higher than average risk of head injury. Symptoms may include unilateral or bilateral headache, periods of confusion with defective memory, misidentification of familiar objects and persons, hallucinations, and epileptic fits. The patient is usually drowsy but the level of consciousness and functional ability of the brain may change from hour to hour. The pupils may vary in size and papilloedema occurs occasionally. Often there are weakness, loss of co-ordination, increased tendon reflexes, clonus and a Babinski sign on the side opposite the subdural haematoma. Cortical sensory deficits may be demonstrable.

Foreign bodies are almost always such an obvious cause of disturbed cerebral function that there is little difficulty in diagnosis. It must be remembered, however, that weeks or months after the impingement of a foreign body on brain tissue, epilepsy and personality changes may appear.

Brain abscess may be due to infection from a nearby, easily detectable source such as otitis media or a compound skull fracture, or from a distant lesion such as bronchiectasis. Occasionally no primary souce of infection can be found. Being a space-occupying lesion, cerebral abscess may give rise to the symptoms and signs discussed under brain tumour. If the abscess ruptures into the subarachnoid space, a superimposed meningitis occurs. In the absence of meningitis, brain abscess causes surprisingly little alteration in temperature, leucocyte count and sedimentation rate.

Tuberculoma is a special type of well-encapsulated, chronic abscess caused by tubercle bacilli. Usually a focus can be discovered, most often pulmonary, but at other times elsewhere, for example, in the genito-urinary or osseous systems. The presence of calcification in a space-occupying lesion visible in skull X-rays should make one consider, among other possibilities, tuberculoma. Tuberculous meningitis is a grave sequel which may occur following spontaneous rupture of a tuberculoma, or as a complication of operative attempts to remove an intracranial tuberculoma.

Gumma is a rare, chronic lesion which appears years after the primary syphilitic infection. A past history of chancre, rash, mucosal ulcers, meningovascular lues, cardio-vascular lues, or treatment because of a positive blood Wasserman test are a few of the clues which help in making a diagnosis. The blood and spinal fluid Wasserman tests are usually positive.

Cysts are rare. Colloid cysts of the third ventricle may cause sudden, severe, recurrent headaches and unconsciousness with or without hypothalamic signs such as hyperthermia. Patients with this condition may be wrongly thought to have idiopathic epilepsy or hysteria.

(b) Obstruction to Cerebrospinal Fluid Circulation

When this occurs, hydrocephalus results, and the cerebral cells are subject to increased mechanical pressure. Mental deficiency is a common sequel to hydrocephalus in childhood. Much less commonly, dementia may develop in adults with lesions such as basilar meningitis or obstructive neoplasms which give rise to hydrocephalus. Ventriculography can provide useful information in localizing the site of obstruction. Blockage of one foramen of Munro produces dilation of only one lateral ventricle. When the aqueduct of Sylvius is obstructed, both lateral ventricles and the third ventricle become enlarged. A blockage at the roof of the fourth ventricle causes dilation of all parts of the ventricular system.

(c) Trauma

Brain injury may be followed by post-traumatic epilepsy, focal neurological disorders, transient acute psychosis, dementia or more subtle personality changes. These sequelae may occur alone or in various combinations. In studying patients suspected of having post-traumatic mental illness, psychological tests, electroencephalographic investigation and X-ray studies, including air encephalography, may help determine whether the brain has been permanently damaged.

Post-traumatic epilepsy appears at varying times after brain injury, up to many months in some instances. Generally speaking, the more severe the injury, the more likely the occurrence of subsequent seizures. If major epileptic seizures are the predominant manifestation, there is usually little diagnostic difficulty. Two other situations may, however, pose a more difficult problem in diagnosis. Firstly, if a grand mal seizure occurs when the patient is alone and confusion or furor follows the convulsion, then the true relationship of the transient mental abnormality to epilepsy may be overlooked. Secondly, the only manifestation of epilepsy may be psychomotor attacks with bizarre behaviour and thought disturbances.

After head injury, behaviour disorders consisting of swings of mood, impulsiveness, outbursts of temper, nervousness, inability to concentrate and a self-centred attitude are common. It is uncertain whether this syndrome is purely psychogenic or not.

REFERENCES

(a) *Space-Occupying Lesions*

(i) *Tumour*

CHAMBERS, W. T.: Misconceptions leading to delay in the diagnosis of intracranial space-taking lesions, Postgrad. Med. 13:405, May 1953.

GOTTESFELD, B. H.: The masking of brain tumors by mental disease, Digest Neurol. & Psychiat. Series XIII: 109, Feb. 1945.

NEWMANN, M. A.: Periventricular diffuse pinealoma, J. Nerv. & Ment. Dis. 121:193, March 1955.

OPPLER, W.: Manic psychosis in a case of parasagittal meningioma, Arch. Neurol. & Psychiat. 64:417, Sept. 1950.

RASKIN, N.: Intracranial neoplasms in psychiatric patients, Am. J. Psychiat. 112:481, Jan. 1956.

SPROFKIN, B. E. and SCIARRA, D.: Korsakoff's psychosis associated with cerebral tumours, Neurology 2:427, Sept.-Oct. 1952.

WHITE, J. C. and COBB, S.: Psychological changes associated with giant pituitary neoplasms, Arch. Neurol. & Psychiat. 74:383, Oct. 1955.

WILLIAMS, M. and PENNYBACKER, J.: Memory disturbances in third ventricle tumours, J. Neurol. Neurosurg. & Psychiat. 17:115, May 1954.

(ii) *Subdural haematoma*

CLARKE, E. and COOPER, R.: Chronic subdural haematoma: Mental change as the principal clinical feature, Lancet 266:1260, June 19, 1954.

FLEISS, A. N.: Psychiatric manifestations of chronic subdural haematomas, Psychiat. Quart. 19:187, April 1945.

LEVIN, S.: Psychomotor epilepsy as a manifestation of subdural haematoma, Am. J. Psychiat. 107:501, Jan. 1951.

(c) *Trauma*

CRITCHLEY, M.:Medical aspects of boxing, particularly from a neurological standpoint, Brit. M.J. 2:357, Feb 16, 1957.

JARVIE, H. F.: Frontal lobe wounds causing disinhibition, J. Neurol. Neurosurg. & Psychiat. 17:14, Feb. 1954.

KAUFMAN, I. C. and WALKER, A. E.: The electroencephalogram after head injury, J. Nerv. & Ment. Dis. 109:383, May 1949.

NOYES, A. P.: Modern Clinical Psychiatry, ed. 4, Philadelphia, W. B. Saunders Co., 1953, chapter 11.

RICHARDSON, J. C.: Post-traumatic cerebral syndromes, Canad. M.A.J. 64:414, May 1951.

STRITCH, S. J.: Diffuse degeneration of the cerebral white matter in severe dementia following head injury, J. Neurol. Neurosurg. & Psychiat. 19:163, Aug. 1956.

CHAPTER VI

Infections

(a) *Primarily Affecting the Central Nervous System*

(i) Meningococci and pneumococci are the organisms most commonly responsible for *pyogenic meningitis.* Other bacteria include staphylococci, Friedlander's bacilli, streptococci, b. proteus, b. pyocyaneus and b. influenzae.

The illness may arise without any evidence of an antecedent focus of infection outside the nervous system or it may be secondary to such conditions as pharyngitis, sinusitis, otitis media, lung abscess, bronchiectasis or sub-acute bacterial endocarditis. Spread of infection may occur by direct extension through portions of the skull or via the blood stream.

The symptoms are well known and will only be briefly mentioned. The onset is usually quite sudden so that within a relatively few hours the patient is seriously ill. Headache, stiff neck, backache, drowsiness, chills and fever, delirium and maniacal behaviour are the main manifestations. Convulsions may occur. Focal neurological signs may be found with extra-ocular muscle palsy being commonest. If a rash is seen, one thinks of meningococcal infection. The temperature and white blood count are elevated. Blood cultures should be taken because the organism is often circulating in the blood stream. The cerebrospinal fluid is under increased pressure, usually appears turbid or even purulent, contains many polymorphonuclear leucocytes, up to 10,000 or more per c. mm., an increased protein concentration and decreased glucose concentration. Smears and cultures must be made to identify the organism and determine its sensitivity to antibacterial drugs. Treatment should, however, be started immediately without awaiting the results of culture.

Tuberculous meningitis, a less acute disease, may be part of a widespread miliary infection or it may be secondary to focal lesions, distant, as in the case of pulmonary tuberculosis, or nearby, in the case of vertebral involvement.

Headache and increasing drowsiness progressing to coma are common symptoms. Symptoms of a confusional state may be conspicuous and precede symptoms and signs of meningeal irritation. Stiff neck and Kernig's sign are usually present. The cerebrospinal fluid which usually appears clear contains excessive lymphocytes up to several hundred or more per c. mm., and in most cases there is a decrease in chloride to less than 600 mg. per 100 ml. Tubercle bacilli can often be demonstrated, the best method being examination of the pellicle which forms when the cerebrospinal fluid is allowed to stand for several hours.

Syphilitic meningtitis occurs in the secondary or tertiary stages of the disease, but is rarely encountered nowadays. The cerebrospinal fluid gives a positive Wasserman test and contains an increased number of lymphocytes.

(ii) Following vaccination with vaccinia virus, or infection with mumps, measles or chickenpox, a rather brief *encephalitis* may occur. Epidemics of encephalitis have resulted from infection with the Japanese encephalitis type B and St. Louis type viruses, as well as the viruses of equine encephalitis. Encephalomyelitis may complicate infectious mononucleosis. It is probable that other organisms, as yet eluding isolation, produce the same clinical syndrome of fever, headache, photophobia, delirium and perhaps meningismus because patients with such findings are encountered fairly often.

Encephalitis lethargica may be followed by permanent disturbances of cerebral function. Behaviour disorders in the form of tantrums and impulsive, irresponsible outbursts can occur, more commonly in children. Years after the acute attack of encephalitis, Parkinsonism may appear and gradually increase in severity. Accompanying the Parkinsonism, occasionally there are oculogyric crises, in which the eyes suddenly rotate, usually in an upward direction. During these episodes, which may last from a minute to an hour or more, some patients experience compulsive, repetitious thought patterns. Many patients with post-encephalitic Parkinsonism are unable to converge the eyes and lack the pupillary reaction to accommodation.

(iii) *General paralysis of the insane* is a chronic organic psychosis due to the invasion of cerebral tissue by the treponema pallidum. Though declining in its incidence, the disease is important because, unless adequately treated, the course is one of increasing mental deterioration ending in death. Mental symptoms run the gamut from mood disorders to paranoia and hallucinations. Judgment fails, indifference about personal cleanliness and the feelings of others becomes evident. One seeks other evidence of syphilis, such as the stigmata of congenital infection—saddle nose, Hutchinson teeth and hepar lobatum, as examples, or in adults a history of exposure, chancre, previous treatment, skin rashes and involvement of mucous membrane. The time between the primary infection and the onset of general paralysis is usually well over five years. Rarely, tertiary luetic lesions in other systems, such as an aneurysm of the thoracic aorta or dilatation of the aortic valve, may coexist. The pupils are usually of the type described by Argyll Robertson. Speech is slurred and the tongue and fingers tremble. Often, pyramidal tract signs, such as spasticity, increased tendon reflexes and positive Babinski responses can be demonstrated. The cerebrospinal fluid Wasserman and the Pandy test for globulin are positive, the colloidal gold curve is characteristic: elevated readings in the first tubes, then falling to 1 or 0 in the later tubes.

(b) Other Infections Sometimes Producing Mental Symptoms

Any acute, severe febrile illness may be accompanied by a brief toxic delirium lasting only hours or days. As a rule, there are no localizing signs of disease of the central nervous system. In addition to these acute infections there are a number of less common infections which may commence with or give rise to symptoms and signs of mental illness. The causative organisms include bacteria (e.g. bacterial endocarditis), spirochaetes (e.g. Weil's disease), protozoan organisms (e.g. malaria and toxoplasmosis) and the larvae of worms (e.g. cysticercosis).

REFERENCES

(a) *Infections with a Predilection for Cerebral Tissues*

(i) *Bacteria*

PAI, M. N.: Personality defects and psychiatric symptoms after cerebrospinal fever in childhood: Meningococcal encephalopathy, J. Ment. Sc. 92:389, April 1946.

WILLIAMS, M. and SMITH, H. V.: Mental disturbances in tuberculous meningitis, J. Neurol. Neurosurg. & Psychiat. 17:173, Aug. 1954.

(ii) *Viruses*

APPELBAUM, E., RACHELSON, M. H. and DOLGOPOL, V. B.: Varicella encephalitis, Am. J. Med. 15:223, Aug. 1953.

ESPIR, M. L. E. and SPALDING, J. M. K.: Three recent cases of encephalitis lethargica, Brit. M. J. 1:1141, May 19, 1956.

FINLEY, K. H., LONGSHORE, W. A., PALMER, R. J., COOK, R. E. and RIGGS, N.: Western equine and St. Louis encephalitis, Neurology 5:223, April 1955.

FULTON, J. S. and BURTON, A. N.: After effects of Western equine encephalomyelitis infection in man, Canad. M.A.J. 69:268, Sept. 1953.

LINDSAY, D. S.: Encephalitis as a psychiatric problem, Am. J. Psychiat. 107:131, Aug. 1950.

MALAMUD, N., HAYMAKER, W. and PINKERTON, H.: Inclusion encephalitis, Am. J. Path. 26:133, Jan. 1950.

MILLER, H. G.: Prognosis of neurologic illness following vaccination against smallpox, Arch. Neurol & Psychiat. 69:695, June 1953.

MITCHELL, W. and PAMPIGLIONE, G.: Neurological and mental complications of rubella, Lancet 267:1250, Dec. 18, 1954.

SMALLPIECE, V. and OUNSTED, C.: Cerebral poliomyelitis in early infancy, J. Neurol. Neurosurg. & Psychiat. 15:13, Feb. 1952.

WOLTMAN, H. W.: Encephalitis: Historical review and perspective, Canad. M.A.J. 77:995, Dec. 1, 1957.

WYATT, N. F.: Japanese B encephalitis: Report of five cases, J. Lab. & Clin. Med. 34:1656, Dec. 1949.

(iii) *General paralysis of the insane*
ESPIR, M. L. E. and WHITTY, C. W. M.: Unusual case of juvenile G.P.I., Brit. M.J. 1:582, March 5, 1955.

(b) *Other Infections Sometimes Producing Mental Symptoms*
ANTEL, J. J., ROME, H. P., GERACI, J. E. and SAYRE, G. P.: Toxic-organic psychosis as a presenting feature in bacterial endocarditis, Proc. Staff Meet. Mayo Clin. 30:45, Feb. 9, 1955.

BICKERSTAFF, E. R.: Cerebral cysticercosis, Brit. M.J. 1:1055, April 30, 1955.

BICKERSTAFF, E. R., CLOAKE, P. C. P., HUGHES, B. and SMITH, W. T.: The racemose form of cerebral cysticercosis, Brain 75:1, 1952.

BREWIS, E. G., NEUBAUER, C. and HURST, E. W.: Another case of louping-ill in man, Lancet 256:689, April 23, 1949.

FREEDMAN, M. J., ODLAND, L. T. and CLEVE, E. A.: Infectious mononucleosis with diffuse involvement of nervous system, Arch. Neurol. & Psychiat. 69:49, Jan. 1953.

GRIFFITH, G.: Neurologic complications of some infectious diseases, Edinburgh M.J. 59:492, Oct. 1952.

KAPLAN, L. I., FLICKER, D. J., BECKER, F. T. and READ, H. S.: Acute psychosis following therapeutic malaria in a case of neuro-syphilis, J. Nerv. & Ment. Dis. 102:285, Sept. 1945.

KASS, E. H., ANDRUS, S. B., ADAMS, R. D., TURNER, F. C. and FELDMAN, H. A.: Toxoplasmosis in the human adult, Arch. Int. Med. 89:759, May 1952.

KERNOHAN, R. J.: Atypical Weil's disease, Brit. M.J. 1:1342, June 9, 1956.

OWEN, T. and LENCZNER, M.: Generalized cysticercosis with cere-bral infestation, Canad. M.A.J. 75:213, Aug. 1, 1956.

REAM, C. R. and HESSING, J. W.: Infectious mononucleosis encepha-litis: Case report, Ann. Int. Med. 41:1231, Dec. 1954.

ROSENBLUM, M. J., MASLAND, R. L. and HARRELL, G. T.: Residual effects of rickettsial disease on the central nervous system, Arch. Int. Med. 90:444, Oct. 1952.

SCOTT, R. A., JOHNSON, R. E. and HOLZMAN, D.: Trichinosis with neurologic and mental manifestations, New England J. Med. 247:512, Oct. 2, 1952.

THOMPSON, T. E., JR. and MILLER, K. F.: Cat scratch encephalitis, Ann. Int. Med. 39:146, July 1953.

THORLING, L.: Neurological complications in acute infectious hepa-titis, Acta med. scandinav. 137:322, 1950.

CHAPTER VII

Intoxications

(*a*) *Exogenous Intoxications*

The aetiological classification presented in an earlier part of the manual gives a practical grouping of the substances responsible for *exogenous* intoxications. The list of medicinal and occupational compounds capable of producing toxic psychoses increases so rapidly from year to year that it is extremely difficult to give a comprehensive tabulation. Here is one place above all others where the alert physician can make appropriate inquiries leading to detection of the toxic substance. He must be willing to question employers and fellow employees, plant doctors, relatives, family doctors and druggists in his search to discover the cause.

As a rule, the illness is of fairly sudden onset and of brief duration. Many of the intoxicants rapidly produce profound metabolic changes which incapacitate the patient. If the intake is excessive, death may occur, but usually recovery takes place in a short time. The patient who becomes ill after ingesting a drug may have an idiosyncracy to a therapeutic dose or he may have taken an excessive amount. On occasion, cardiac, hepatic or renal insufficiency is present with consequent impaired excretion of the toxic substance.

The mental changes range from mild anxiety to florid psychotic symptoms, for example, excitement, disorientation, paranoid states, auditory and visual hallucinations. The mental changes have little specific diagnostic value, except to suggest an organic factor. In determining the responsible agent, careful inquiry into drug treatments and into exposure to toxins at home or at work is the most important investigative approach. Sedatives, stimulants, muscle relaxants and various tonics are so often used in treating mentally ill patients that the possibility of a coexisting drug intoxication should always be kept in mind.

Physical examination may reveal other signs of reaction to toxic materials such as fever, skin rash, lead or bismuth lines and neuropathy, the exact signs depending in part on the responsible agent.

The laboratory can provide great help in certain of these intoxications. Information about the submission of specimens for such tests can be found in chapter xv. The doctor should obtain such samples as soon after the onset of the illness as possible because most of these substances are rapidly excreted.

A few of the distinctive features of some of the toxic reactions are worthy of mention. *Bromides*, particularly in elderly, nervous people who sleep poorly may produce a delirium in which auditory hallucinations are common. Some alcoholic or barbiturate habitués change their drug habit to bromide ingestion and become psychotic. The serum level at the onset of the delirium is nearly always 100 mg. per 100 ml. or higher. Not all patients with high serum concentrations of bromide develop mental symptoms, there being marked differences in individual response to the drug. *Barbiturates* are used medicinally in enormous quantities and are often taken for suicidal reasons. When a large amount is ingested, coma ensues. When they are taken in smaller amounts over a long period of time, chronic intoxication with mental clouding, impairment of judgment and apathy about personal appearance may appear in conjunction with slurred speech, tremulousness and ataxia. If bromides, barbiturates or alcohol be suddenly discontinued by persons accustomed to excessive amounts over a long period, rather florid symptoms may develop, such as grand mal seizures, anxiety, hallucinations and paranoid states.

Alcohol: *Delirium tremens* is probably the commonest type of delirium apart from acute alcoholic intoxication. As a rule, the diagnosis is quickly made, all doctors and most lay people being familiar with the condition. However, if the patient is not known to be an alcoholic, then the diagnosis may be unsuspected at first. It is important to appreciate that some people are able to consume large amounts of alcohol daily for long periods without their family, their friends or themselves realizing that they are addicted to alcohol and without their efficiency as a worker being so seriously impaired that they have to give up their job. Such individuals may deny drinking excessively and their relatives and friends may corroborate the story. After an unusually heavy drinking bout, or if the intake of alcohol suddenly stops because of ill-health or injury, the patient may suffer from delirium tremens with the usual features of anxiety, marked restlessness, tremulousness and the characteristic hallucinations. Also, during this period of withdrawal from alcohol, the patient may have one or more generalized epileptic seizures. The course of the illness is well known, patients usually recovering from the acute delirium within a few days, although rarely the illness may develop into a Korsakoff's psychosis (see p. 18).

It happens, not uncommonly, that patients who have consumed large quantities of alcohol for a long time display a gradual deterioration of personality with features of dementia. Sometimes, but not always, cerebral atrophy may be demonstrated by air encephalography. Ataxia and inco-ordination occasionally accompany the dementia in which case one may see signs of cerebellar atrophy in the air encephalogram. Excessive intake of alcohol over a period of years would seem to release a syndrome, designated alcoholic hallucinosis. The characteristic features are usually auditory hallucinations related to underlying personality conflicts and occurring in a clear sensorium. Fear and apprehension are usually present but there is no disorientation. On recovery, the patient can recall the steps in the illness without difficulty. Since this pattern lacks most of the fundamental features of an organic psychosis it is usually considered a functional mental illness precipitated by alcoholic excess. Recovery commonly occurs in a matter of weeks but occasionally the illness merges into a schizophrenic pattern.

Benzedrine is used as a nasal inhalant for nasal congestion and in the form of tablets to defer sleepiness, particularly in students and orchestra members. Obese persons use the drug to depress the appetite. Benzedrine may produce a nervous, hyper-excitable state or a florid psychosis often with para-noidal features; in very large doses benzedrine may give rise to coma and death. *Arsenicals* are used less frequently now as insecticides or medicinally, but arsenical poisoning is occasionally seen. Certain features of arsenical poisoning are: the hyperkeratotic lesions of the palms and soles, peripheral neuritis, agranulocytosis and aplastic anaemia. Arsenic can be detected, long after ingestion, by analysis of the hair and nail clippings. Intravenously administered arsenicals, especially when given in frequent, large doses, may produce a severe, sometimes fatal, acute encephalopathy with delirium, headache, papilloedema and focal neurological signs. *Mercurial compounds* may produce salivism, chronic irritability and occasionally psychosis. *Thiocyanates* are still occasionally prescribed for hypertensive patients. Psychosis is a common complication if serum levels of the drug are not followed. When the serum concentration exceeds 12 mg. per 100 ml., mental changes may be seen. Skin rashes, aching of bones, and depression of the bone marrow are some of the other undesirable side-effects. It seems well established that the *rauwolfia compounds*, of which reserpine is one of the most widely used, induce a state of depression in some patients. The clinical picture mimics closely the depression of involutional melancholia and is surprisingly devoid of evidences of organic intellectual impairment such as one sees in most other drug psychoses. Although the mental state lacks the features of a dementia or a delirium, we include the condition in the organic psychoses because the drug appears to play a major part in producing the mental illness. *Antihistamine compounds* are widely used for hay-fever, for urticaria, and (despite their lack of value) for the common cold. Acute intoxications with ataxia and delirium as features may occur with quite small doses of these drugs in certain susceptible persons. *Cocaine* induces a cutaneous paraesthesia as if the insects were burrowing through the skin. *Lead* poisoning usually results from exposure in factories or the home workshop. Bouts of intestinal colic and severe constipation occur, sometimes over a period of many months. Some patients convulse and become delirious. A blue-grey lead line can usually be seen near the teeth. Lead is a renal tubular toxin capable of producing nephrosis. Anaemia is usually present and the blood smear studied with special stains will show many stippled red cells. The blood and urine contain abnormally high amounts of lead.

(b) Endogenous Intoxications

We refer to conditions such as uraemia and liver failure. The substances (and it seems likely that there are such substances) responsible for the clinical picture of uraemia and liver failure have not been identified with certainty.

Uraemia has many causes which may be conveniently classified as prerenal, renal or postrenal. Prerenal causes refer to all conditions which reduce renal blood flow to the point where renal function is impaired. Examples are severe hypotension due to trauma, Addison's disease and burns, or dehydration due to prolonged vomiting or diarrhoea. The renal conditions are diffuse kidney diseases such as glomerulonephritis, pyelonephritis and nephrosclerosis. Obstructive lesions of the renal pelves, ureters and urethra due to conditions such as tumours, strictures or prostatic hypertrophy make up the postrenal group. Clinical evidences of renal insufficiency include oliguria, muscle twitching, convulsions, coma, delirium or lesser degrees of mental confusion. The level of non-protein nitrogen and the concentration of blood urea are increased and in most instances the urine contains albumin, cells and casts.

Hepatic insufficiency may be present in any disease which causes diffuse damage to liver cells. Intrahepatic conditions include portal cirrhosis, juvenile cirrhosis, biliary cirrhosis and subacute yellow atrophy. Obstructive lesions such as a stone in the common bile duct or carcinoma either of bile ducts or the head of the pancreas may produce obstructive biliary cirrhosis with hepatic failure. One should appreciate that a patient with severe hepatic insufficiency need not be jaundiced. Helpful in substantiating a diagnosis of liver disease are telangiectases, xanthomata, "liver palms," ascites and evidences of portal obstruction such as oesophageal varices, haemorrhoids or a caput Medusae. The mental state may be one of drowsiness progressing later to coma, and agitation with outbursts of crying and mournful shouting. An attitude of flexor rigidity may appear, the limbs move in a "flapping" manner, and Babinski signs are often present. Valuable laboratory tests include those for bile and urobilin in the urine, the van den Bergh, cephalin cholesterol flocculation and serum protein determinations. The measurement of the excretion of bromsulphthalein is a more delicate test of liver function. Because liver disease severe enough to produce jaundice is always accompanied by decreased excretion of bromsulphthalein, the test only gives useful information in the absence of jaundice.

REFERENCES

(a) *Exogenous Intoxications*
   (i) *Medication*
   LEVIN, M.: The frequency of drug psychoses, Am. J. Psychiat. 107:128, Aug. 1950.
   ——— Toxic delirium precipitated by admission to the hospital: With remarks on the diagnosis of incipient drug delirium, J. Nerv. & Ment. Dis. 116:210, Sept. 1952.
   WIKLER, A.: Mechanism of action of drugs that modify personality function, Am. J. Psychiat. 108:590, Feb. 1952.

   (1) *Sedatives*
   GAYLE, R. F., JR. and GEE, G. L., JR.: Clinical aspects of barbiturate intoxication, Virginia M. Month. 80:560, Oct. 1953.

HEWITT, R. T.: A psychosis with barbiturate withdrawal, J. Nerv. & Ment. Dis. 112:526, Dec. 1950.

LEVIN, M.: Bromide delirium with unusual course, Am. J. Psychiat. 110:130, Aug. 1953.

MARLEY, E. and CHAMBERS, J. S. W.: Toxic effects and side-effects of methylpentynol, Brit. M.J. 2:1467, Dec. 22, 1956.

MORGAN, N. C.: Psychosis resulting from barbiturate withdrawal, J.A.M.A. 149:759, June 21, 1952.

(2) *Stimulants*

CARR, R. B.: Acute psychotic reaction after inhaling methylamphetamine, Brit. M.J. 1:1476, June 26, 1954.

CHAPMAN, A. H.: Paranoid psychoses associated with amphetamine usage, Am. J. Psychiat. 111:43, July 1954.

HERMAN, M. and NAGLER, S. H.: Psychoses due to amphetamine, J. Nerv. & Ment. Dis. 120:268, Sept.-Oct. 1954.

KJAER-LARSEN, J.: Delirious psychosis and convulsions due to megimide, Lancet 271:967, Nov. 10, 1956.

(3) *Chemotherapeutic and antibiotic agents*

COHEN, S. B.: Psychosis resulting from penicillin hypersensitivity, Am. J. Psychiat. 111:699, March 1955.

CRANE, G. E.: The psychiatric side-effects of iproniazid, Am. J. Psychiat. 112:494, Jan. 1956.

HALPERN, L., STREIFLER, M. and LAZSLO, L.: The electrical activity of the brain in a case of atabrine psychosis, Am. J. Psychiat. 110:366, Nov. 1953.

HITCH, J. M.: Neurotoxic symptoms following use of asterol dihydrochloride: Report of three cases, J.A.M.A. 150:1004, Nov. 8, 1952.

HUNTER, R. A.: Confusional psychosis with residual organic cerebral impairment following isoniazid therapy, Lancet 263:960, Nov. 15, 1952.

MCCONNELL, R. B. and CHEETHAM, H. D.: Acute pellagra during isoniazid therapy, Lancet 263:959, Nov. 15, 1952.

MITCHELL, R. S.: Fatal toxic encephalitis occurring during iproniazid therapy in pulmonary tuberculosis, Ann. Int. Med. 42:417, Feb. 1955.

NEWELL, H. W. and LIDZ, T.: The toxicity of atabrine to the central nervous system, Am. J. Psychiat. 102:805, May 1946.

SHEPPECK, M. L. and WEXBERG, L. E.: Toxic psychoses associated with administration of quinacrine, Arch. Neurol. & Psychiat. 55:489, May 1946.

WILSON, J. W., LEVITT, H., HARRIS, T. L. and HEILIGMAN, E. M.: Toxic encephalopathy occurring during topical therapy with asterol, J.A.M.A. 150:1002, Nov. 8, 1952.

(4) *Hormones*

CLARK, L. D., BAUER, W. and Cobb, S.: Preliminary observations on mental disturbances occurring in patients under therapy with cortisone and ACTH, New England J. Med. 246:205, Feb. 7, 1952.

CLARK, L. D., QUARTON, G. C., COBB, S. and BAUER, W.: Further observations on mental disturbances associated with cortisone and ACTH therapy, New England J. Med. 249:178, July 30, 1953.

GLASER, G. H.: Psychotic reactions induced by corticotrophin (ACTH) and cortisone, Psychosom. Med. 15:280, July-Aug. 1953.

GOOLKER, P. and SCHEIN, J.: Psychic effects of ACTH and cortisone, Psychosom. Med. 15:589, Nov.-Dec. 1953.

HOEFER, P. F. A. and GLASER, G. H.: Effects of pituitary adrenocorticotrophic hormone (ACTH) therapy: Electroencephalographic and neuropsychiatric changes in fifteen patients, J.A.M.A. 143:620, June 17, 1950.

ROME, H. P. and BRACELAND, F. J.: Psychological response to corticotropin, cortisone and related steroid substances, J.A.M.A. 148:27, Jan. 5, 1952.

(5) *Hypotensor drugs*

ACHOR, R. W. P., HANSON, N. O. and GIFFORD, R. W., JR.: Hypertension treated with rauwolfia serpentina (whole root) and with reserpine: Controlled study disclosing occasional severe depression, J.A.M.A. 159:841, Oct. 29, 1955.

BARNETT, H. J. M., JACKSON, M. V. and SPAULDING, W. B.: Thiocyanate psychosis, J.A.M.A. 147:1554, Dec. 15, 1951.

DANZIG, L. E. and KRINGEL, A. J.: Use of the artificial kidney in treatment of thiocyanate psychosis, J.A.M.A. 158:560, June 18, 1955.

DOMZALSKI, C. A., KOLB, L. C. and HINES, E. A., JR.: Delirious reactions secondary to thiocyanate therapy of hypertension, Proc. Staff Meet. Mayo Clin. 28:272, May 6, 1953.

FREIS, E. D.: Mental depression in hypertensive patients treated for long periods with large doses of reserpine, New England J. Med. 251:1006, Dec. 16, 1954.

LEMIEUX, G., DAVIGNON, A. and GENEST, J.: Depressive states during rauwolfia therapy for arterial hypertension, Canad. M.A.J. 74:522, April 1, 1956.

MOSER, M., SYNER, J., MALITZ, S. and MATTINGLY, T. W.: Acute psychosis as a complication of hydralazine therapy in essential hypertension, J.A.M.A. 152:1329, Aug. 1, 1953.

MULLER, J. C., PRYOR, W. W., GIBBONS, J. E. and ORGAIN, E. S.: Depression and anxiety occurring during rauwolfia therapy, J.A.M.A. 159:836, Oct. 29, 1955.

SCHROEDER, H. A. and PERRY, H. M.: Psychosis apparently produced by reserpine, J.A.M.A. 159: 839, Oct. 29, 1955.

SMITH, T. P.: Acute hallucinatory episode following hexamethonium bromide, Brit. M.J. 1:1088, May 12, 1956.

(6) *Miscellaneous*

BETHELL, M. F.: Toxic psychosis caused by "Preludin," Brit. M.J. 1:30, Jan. 5, 1957.

FISKE, D.: "Psychotic reaction" to tetraethylthiuram disulfide (antabuse) therapy, J.A.M.A. 150:1110, Nov. 15, 1952.

GROISSER, V. W.: Atropine poisoning: Report of two cases, Ann. Int. Med. 44:1020, May 1956.

MACKLIN, E. A., SIMON, A. and HAMILTON, G. H.: Pyschotic reactions in problem drinkers treated with disulfiram (antabuse), Arch. Neurol. & Psychiat. 69:415, April 1953.

PIERIK, M. G.: Acute hallucinosis secondary to pagitane hydrochloride administration, New England J. Med. 251:1058, Dec. 23, 1954.

PORTEOUS, H. B. and ROSS, D. N.: Mental symptoms in Parkinsonism following benzhexol hydrochloride therapy, Brit. M.J. 2:138, July 21, 1956.

TODD, J.: Trichlorethylene poisoning with paranoid psychosis and Lilliputian hallucination, Brit. M.J. 1:439, Feb. 20, 1954.

WALDMAN, S. and PELNER, L.: Toxic psychosis due to overdosage with prophenpyridamine (trimeton), J.A.M.A. 143:1334, Aug. 12, 1950.

YAPALATER, A. R. and ROCKWELL, F. V.: Toxic psychosis due to prophenpyridamine (trimeton), J.A.M.A. 143:428, June 3, 1950.

(ii) *Self-administered*

BENNETT, I. L., JR., CARY, F. H., MITCHELL, G. L., JR. and COOPER, M. N.: Acute methyl alcohol poisoning, Medicine 32:431, Dec. 1953.

LEMERE, F.: The nature and significance of brain damage from alcoholism, Am. J. Psychiat. 113:361, Oct. 1956.

SKILLICORN, S. A.: Presenile cerebellar ataxia in chronic alcoholics, Neurology 5:527, Aug. 1955.

THOMPSON, G. N. (Editor): Alcoholism, Springfield, Illinois, Charles C. Thomas, 1956.

TUMARKIN, B., WILSON, J. D. and SNYDER, G.: Cerebral atrophy due to alcoholism in young adults, U.S. Armed Forces M.J. 6:67, Jan. 1955.

(iii) *Occupational*

BELKNAP, E. L.: Differential diagnosis of lead poisoning, J.A.M.A. 139:818, March 26, 1949.

HUNTER, D.: The Diseases of Occupations, ed. 2, London, The English Universities Press Ltd., 1957, pp. 568–571.

KLEINFELD, M. and TABERSHAW, I. R.: Carbon disulfide poinsoning, J.A.M.A. 159:677, Oct. 15, 1955.

MACRAE, M. M.: A case of methyl chloride poisoning, Brit. M.J. 1:1134, May 15, 1954.

STEVENS, H. and FORSTER, F. M.: Effect of carbon tetrachloride on the nervous system, Arch. Neurol. & Psychiat. 70:635, Nov. 1953.

WALKER, G. and BOYD, P. R.: Tetraethyl lead poisoning, Lancet 263:467, Sept. 6, 1952.

(b) *Endogenous Intoxications*

BAKER, A. B. and KNUTSON, J.: Psychiatric aspects of uraemia, Am. J. Psychiat. 102:683, March 1946.

JEFFERSON, M.: Mental confusion after porto-caval anastomosis, Brit. M.J. 1:786, March 26, 1955.

HAVENS, L. L. and CHILD, C. G. III: Recurrent psychosis associated with liver disease and elevated blood ammonia, New England J. Med. 252:756, May 5, 1955.

HURWITZ, L. H. and ALLISON, R. S.: Recurring mental confusion after porto-caval anastomosis, Brit. M.J. 1:387, Feb. 12, 1955.

SHERLOCK, S., SUMMERSKILL, W. H. J., WHITE, L. P. and PHEAR, E. A.: Portal-systemic encephalopathy—neurological complications of liver disease, Lancet 267:453, Sept. 4, 1954.

CHAPTER VIII

Degenerations of Cerebral Tissue

We are using the word "degenerations" in a broad sense to include a number of diseases of obscure aetiology. Under this heading will be found conditions in which there is degeneration of cells of the cerebral cortex, of cells in deeper parts of the brain and of the myelin surrounding axonal processes. Thus we include certain demyelinating diseases in this group. Because there is little precise knowledge of the causes of the cellular dysfunction in these diseases, we have not attempted to classify them further.

Huntington's chorea is a hereditary disease which usually first manifests itself between the ages of twenty and fifty. The cardinal features are a combination of progressive mental deterioration, leading to severe dementia, associated with chorea. Early in the course of the illness, either the mental impairment or the chorea may dominate the clinical picture, but most patients become severely demented in the later stages of the disease. As is so often the case in diseases which give rise to dementia, the earliest mental changes may be predominantly those found in functional illnesses, such as behaviour disorders or abnormalities of mood. Thus the patient may become depressed before the disease has seemingly progressed very far, or a young adult may exhibit faulty judgment and irresponsible behaviour and be diagnosed as a psychopathic personality before dementia is recognized.

When the chorea is well established, the face and limbs are seen to contort in bizarre grimaces and purposeless, jerky movements. The gait may resemble that of a drunken man trying to dance. As the disease progresses, dysarthria and ataxia may become very marked. The inherited defect is carried by a dominant gene and results in approximately one half the children of an affected parent becoming afflicted with the disease. Therefore, the taking of a detailed family history is of the greatest importance in establishing a diagnosis of Huntington's chorea. It should be noted, however, that patients are sometimes seen in whom the most searching inquiries of relatives fail to reveal a family history of the disease and yet the patient has the typical clinical features. In such cases the family may be concealing the true facts, or the patient may have been an illegitimate child whose father is not known, or, as sometimes seems more probable, the disease is arising afresh as a mutation.

Alzheimer's disease and *Pick's disease* are presenile dementias which are often difficult to distinguish clinically. In fact no useful, practical purpose is served by attempting to make the clinical distinction, for the similarities of the two diseases are more striking than the differences. Both tend to have their onset between the ages of forty and sixty. It is not uncommon to find that other members of the family have been similarly affected. The cardinal feature of these diseases is a slowly progressive dementia which is frequently quite profound within two or three years of the onset. Patients often exhibit marked changes in behaviour and mood. Before the dementia is of severe degree, these changes in personality may dominate the clinical picture with the result that mistaken diagnoses, for example, involutional melancholia, are sometimes made. Before noticing any intellectual impairment, the family may observe that the patient has become facetious, unusually jocular with inappropriate laughing, or subject to unexpected bouts of irritability or vindictiveness. There may be a loss of finer sensibilities, carelessness in housekeeping, indifference about personal appearance and a lack of modesty. Particularly if the patient is well educated and well spoken, he may rather cleverly conceal the evidences of dementia by giving plausible reasons for his lapses of memory, mistakes in calculation or inability to find his way about the neighbourhood.

The patterns of intellectual impairment vary a good deal in patients with well-established presenile dementia. Thus one patient may have the greatest difficulty in doing simple arithmetical sums but is able to maintain a fair grasp of current affairs. Another may calculate fairly well but be quite unable to draw or understand a simple map of the streets near his home. In the early stages of the illness the clinical evidence of dementia may be equivocal; in studying such cases an experienced clinical psychologist using a battery of special tests may give considerable help. These tests sometimes reveal mental changes of diagnostic importance such as memory defects, inability to learn unfamiliar material or an inability to solve problems involving spatial relationships.

Patients with presenile dementia also vary considerably in their degree of insight. Commonly, the patient has little or no awareness of the severity of the loss of his mental powers, but occasionally a patient will be conscious of his own decline and become severely depressed about his increasing intellectual deficiences.

Physical examination may reveal increased movements of the limbs and head; some patients have abrupt, jerky movements and may move their hands, limbs and face continuously in a restless fashion. Increased muscle tone and a loss of facial expression occur commonly. In the later stages, strong pouting and grasp reflexes can frequently be elicited. Air encephalography often reveals ventricular dilatation. However, in individual cases there may be little or no correlation between the severity of the dementia and the degree of ventricular dilatation and widening of sulci, some severely demented patients having remarkably little radiological evidence of cerebral atrophy.

Alzheimer's disease tends to involve the brain more extensively than Pick's disease so that in the former condition epileptic fits and other neurological disorders such as aphasia and hemiparesis are more likely to occur. It is in such cases that difficulties may arise in excluding other diagnostic possibilities such as brain tumour or cerebral vascular disease. Generally speaking, the presenile dementias run a progressive course with increasing mental and physical deterioration, marked loss of weight and death occurring within five to ten years of the onset.

Senile cerebral atrophy with psychosis is a common disease of advanced age. Early in the illness minor changes are noted: memory loss for recent events, irritability, indifference about appearance and a selfish petulance. Over a few years, the mental deterioration progresses to marked dementia with or without other features such as agitation, depression or paranoia.

Disseminated sclerosis has two distinctive characteristics: it is not a steadily progressive disease and the lesions are always disseminated. Because symptoms wax and wane, and because paraesthesias may be present without accompanying objective physical findings, a diagnosis of hysteria is often made early in the disease. The onset is usually between ages fifteen and forty. The isolated, scattered lesions of the central nervous system usually alter the functions of cranial nerves, long tracts and the cerebellum. Among the many neurological abnormalities which may be found, particular mention should be made of retrobulbar neuritis resulting in pallor of the temporal portions of the optic discs, loss of abdominal reflexes and disturbances of bladder function. A frank psychosis is rare but one often observes blunting of finer sensibilities, disregard for the seriousness of the neurological disease, unnatural euphoria or moderate intellectual impairment. In about half the cases there is a moderate elevation of protein in the cerebrospinal fluid and the colloidal gold curve may be of the paretic type.

It is debatable whether disseminated sclerosis should be included in an aetiological classification of organic psychoses. According to the definition we have chosen, an organic psychosis is any mental illness in which a physical factor disturbing the function of cerebral cells plays a major role in causing the mental illness and in most cases produces features of delirium or dementia eventually. In disseminated sclerosis there is often undoubted involvement of cerebral tissue and frequently the mental state is altered from normal. However, the degree of alteration is usually not great and delirium or dementia rarely if ever occurs. Because it is common for patients with disseminated sclerosis to be admitted to psychiatric wards with a diagnosis of hysteria, and because the possibility of disseminated sclerosis arises in the differential diagnosis of certain patients with mental abnormalities and neurological findings, we have elected to include this brief reference to the disease.

Schilder's disease or periaxialis encephalitis diffusa is a demyelinating process usually beginning at the occipital poles and extending forward continuously to reach the frontal poles. The disease which affects children and young adults is characterized by blindness, convulsions and dementia. More focal neurological signs like spastic paralysis also occur.

Tuberous sclerosis (epiloia) is a sclerosing disease of myelin in which scattered focal lesions, likened to drops of candlewax, appear in the brain. A distinctive feature, usually present, is a facial or more widespread skin rash called adenoma sebaceum in which swollen sebaceous glands appear as small bumps particularly on the nose and cheeks. Epilepsy and mental defect are the main results of the involvement of the brain. Tuberous sclerosis sometimes has a familial occurrence. Some patients have fibromata under the nails, others have changes in the lungs and some have tumours of the heart and kidney.

Friedreich's ataxia is a hereditary disease of the nervous system which may give rise to impairment of mental ability. Patients often have associated anomalies, the most frequent being pes cavus and scoliosis. The degenerative process affects the posterior columns of the spinal cord to the greatest extent but the spinocerebellar and pyramidal tracts may be involved. Nystagmus and dysarthria are present in many cases. Cardiac involvement occurs with sufficient frequency to warrant electrocardiographic examination of anyone suspected of having the disease; defects of conduction, such as heart block, are often revealed. The onset is usually in childhood or early adult life and the disease tends to progress slowly over a number of years.

REFERENCES

BORNSTEIN, S. and JERVIS, G. A.: Presenile dementia of the Jakob type, Arch. Neurol. & Psychiat. 74:598, Dec. 1955.

EWALT, J. R. and HANES, L. C.: Cortical atrophy as etiological factor in certain types of mental disorders, Texas Rep. Biol. & Med. 6:354, Fall 1948.

JONES, D. P. and NEVIN, S.: Rapidly progressive cerebral degeneration (subacute vascular encephalopathy) with mental disorder, focal disturbances and myoclonic epilepsy, J. Neurol. Neurosurg. & Psychiat. 17:148, May 1954.

MEYER, A., LEIGH, D. and BAGG, C. E.: A rare presenile dementia associated with cortical blindness (Heidenhain's syndrome), J. Neurol. Neurosurg. & Psychiat. 17:129, May 1954.

NEUMANN, M. A. and COHN, R.: Incidence of Alzheimer's disease in a large mental hospital, Arch. Neurol. & Psychiat. 69:615, May 1953.

PARR, D.: Diagnostic problems in pre-senile dementia illustrated by a case of Alzheimer's disease proven histologically during life, J. Ment. Sc. 101:387, April 1955.

PLEYDELL, M. J.: Huntington's chorea in Northamptonshire, Brit. M.J. 2:1121, Nov. 13, 1954.

POLATIN, P., HOCH, P. H., HORWITZ, W. A. and ROIZIN, L.: Presenile psychosis: Report of two cases with brain biopsy studies, Am. J. Psychiat. 105:96, Aug. 1948.

RASKIN, N. and EHRENBERG, R.: Senescence, senility, and Alzheimer's disease, Am. J. Psychiat. 113:133, Aug. 1956.

ROTHSCHILD, D.: Pathologic changes in senile psychoses and their psychobiologic significance, Am. J. Psychiat. 93:757, Jan. 1937.

SJÖGREN, T., SJÖGREN, H. and LINDGREN, A. G. H.: Morbus Alzheimer and morbus Pick, Acta Psychiat. et Neurol. Scandinav. (Supp. 82), 1952.

STERN, K. and REED, G. E.: Presenile dementia (Alzheimer's disease), Am. J. Psychiat. 102:191, Sept. 1945.

TORRENS, J. K. and OTTO, J. L.: Psychoses with multiple sclerosis, Dis. Nerv. System 10:243, Aug. 1949.

CHAPTER IX

Paroxysmal Cerebral Dysrhythmias

The reader may wonder why it is considered necessary to include a discussion of epilepsy in a monograph dealing with organic psychoses. There are, however, a number of ways in which patients who have, or are suspected of having, epilepsy may present problems in diagnosis with regard to the organic syndromes. With the widespread use of electroencephalography it has become commonplace to encounter patients suffering from various so-called functional psychiatric disorders such as psychopathic personality, adolescent behaviour disorder or schizophrenic reaction in whom there are definite abnormalities of the electroencephalogram. Furthermore, some of these patients describe paroxysmal disorders of emotion and thought which closely resemble the descriptions of patients known to have epilepsy due to lesions of the temporal lobes. Surveys of groups of aggressive psychopathic individuals and of patients with schizophrenic disorders, for example, have revealed a higher incidence of abnormal electroencephalograms than in mentally healthy subjects. What these observations mean with regard to the causation of such illnesses is impossible to state with certainty at present. However, from a practical standpoint, the physician often must decide how far he should go in attempting to demonstrate a lesion of the brain and whether anticonvulsant drugs should be used in conjunction with psychotherapy. The fact that most of these patients have no demonstrable cerebral lesions on gross or routine microscopic examination must be balanced against the fact that the occasional patient who has, for example, been treated as a case of adolescent behaviour disorder with outbursts of rage has been found to have a cerebral lesion, the surgical removal of which resulted in a marked improvement in behaviour. Thus, cases of temporal lobe epilepsy have been diagnosed psychoneurosis, defect of personality or functional psychosis for a long time before it was realized that an important factor in the aetiology of the mental disorder was a physiological disturbance of the temporal lobe. Another difficulty may arise in diagnosing the causes of disturbances of the mental state which occur after major epileptic attacks, states which have been variously described by the phrases post-ictal confusion, furor or psychosis, post-ictal automatism or amnesia. The significance of such disorders may fail to be appreciated if the patient is not a known epileptic and if no reliable witness observed the convulsion.

The relationship between epilepsy and functional mental illnesses is further complicated by the following possibilities. Occasionally an emotional upset will precipitate an epileptic seizure. If this fact is not appreciated, the patient's condition may be considered to be entirely of psychogenic origin and no attempt made to investigate the epileptic component. Furthermore, it is not rare for epilepsy and hysteria (or other forms of functional mental illness) to coexist in the same person. The hysterical attacks may be so obvious and may so overshadow the epileptic attacks that a diagnosis of epilepsy is not seriously entertained.

The different types of lesions which may give rise to epilepsy are so numerous that no attempt will be made to list them here. Instead it may be stated that the majority of the disorders listed in the Aetiological Classification of Organic Psychoses (chapter II) may, in certain patients, give rise to epileptic attacks. Thus a useful though non-specific clue to the presence of an organic factor affecting the function of cerebral cells in a mentally ill patient is the occurrence of epileptic phenomena. If these phenomena include symptoms or signs of focal cerebral disturbance, then clinical study of the attacks will help to reveal which part of the brain is affected. Particular attention should be paid to the patient's description of the aura, because sensory disturbances, such as paraesthesias in one hand or one side of the face, may be important indications of a focal lesion of the brain. The manner in which the convulsion begins may also be indicative of a local abnormality, for example, a generalized convulsion may be preceded by clonic contractions of the muscles of one limb.

It might seem a simple matter to determine whether or not a patient has been having grand mal convulsions. However, unless the attacks have been observed by a doctor or some other reliable witness, diagnosis may be difficult. Nocturnal convulsions should be strongly suspected if others hear the brief cry at the onset of the fit or the sound of the patient threshing about in bed. If, in addition, there is evidence of bed-wetting and tongue-biting as well as a history from the patient that on awakening he felt stiff and ached all over, it is almost certain that a grand mal seizure has occurred.

One should be familiar with the types of epileptic attacks occurring in some patients with lesions of the temporal lobe. Sudden outbursts usually lasting a few minutes may occur without a preceding convulsion. For example, there may be brief spells of purposeless running, or outbursts of temper with physical aggressiveness. In addition to these psychomotor equivalents, patients may experience brief dream-like states with visual or auditory hallucinations, disturbed visual impressions, feelings of unreality, "déjà vu" feelings of having been in exactly the same situation before, gustatory fits in which an evil taste is noted, or olfactory fits in which a foul odour is noted. These sensory experiences may be part of the aura of a convulsion or occur without a subsequent grand mal fit. Disturbances of mood, for example, depression or anxiety, may accompany or follow these attacks. In the investigation of patients suspected of having lesions of the temporal lobes, the use of sphenoidal electroencephalographic leads and demonstration of the temporal horns of the lateral ventricles by air encephalography may provide evidence of a focal lesion. Some patients with epilepsy display evidence of a gradually developing mild to moderate dementia. In these cases, usually the epilepsy has been of many years' duration. The reason for the mental deterioration is not known for certain.

Research in neurophysiology, especially in this area of the epilepsies, has been progressing rapidly in the last few years. One result has been the realization that focal cerebral disturbances are responsible for epilepsy more frequently than was formerly appreciated. The role of electroencephalography has become better defined. In the diagnosis of epilepsy the electroencephalogram is often confirmatory and may disclose a focal disturbance. But it should be remembered, in considering individual patients, that some apparently normal persons have abnormal electroencephalograms and that some epileptic patients have normal tracings between fits. Indeed, frequently the clinician is perplexed in his attempts to evaluate the electro-encephalographer's report of paroxysmal abnormalities suggestive of epilepsy in patients with functional mental illness. It may be difficult or impossible to correlate these findings with the clinical picture. Futhermore, anticonvulsant therapies not infrequently fail to produce a favourable effect on the clinical state.

REFERENCES

Bourne, H.: Acute epileptic dementia: A contribution to the problem of mental deterioration in epileptics, J. Nerv. & Ment. Dis. 122:288, Sept. 1955.

Ervin, F., Epstein, A. W. and King, H. E.: Behaviour of epileptic and nonepileptic patients with "temporal spikes," Arch. Neurol. & Psychiat. 74:488, Nov. 1955.

Falconer, M. A.: Clinical manifestations of temporal lobe epilepsy and their recognition in relation to surgical treatment, Brit. M.J. 2:939, Oct. 23, 1954.

Falconer, M. A. and Pond, D. A. with pathological reports by Meyer, A. and Woolf, A. L.: Temporal lobe epilepsy with personality and behaviour disorders caused by an unusual calcifying lesion (report of two cases in children relieved by temporal lobectomy), J. Neurol. Neurosurg. & Psychiat. 16:234, Nov. 1953.

GALLINEK, A.: Organic sequelae of electric convulsive therapy including facial and body dysgnosias, J. Nerv. & Ment. Dis. 115:377, May 1952.

KARAGULLA, S. and ROBERTSON, E. E.: Psychical phenomena in temporal lobe epilepsy and the psychoses, Brit. M.J. 1:748, March 26, 1955.

LEVIN, S.: Epileptic clouded states—a review of 52 cases, J. Nerv. & Ment. Dis. 116:215, Sept. 1952.

MARTIN, H. L. and McDOWELL, F.: Evaluation of seizures in the adult, Arch. Neurol. & Psychiat. 71:101, Jan. 1954.

MEYER, A., BECK, E. and SHEPHERD, M.: Unusually severe lesions in the brain following status epilepticus, J. Neurol. Neurosurg. & Psychiat. 18:24, Feb. 1955.

MEYER, A., FALCONER, M. A. and BECK, E.: Pathological findings in temporal lobe epilepsy, J. Neurol. Neurosurg. & Psychiat. 17:276, Nov. 1954.

MEYER, V. and YATES, A. J.: Intellectual changes following temporal lobectomy for psychomotor epilepsy, J. Neurol. Neurosurg. & Psychiat. 18:44, Feb. 1955.

MULDER, D. W.: Paroxysmal psychiatric symptoms observed in epilepsy, Proc. Staff Meet. Mayo Clin. 28:31, Jan. 28, 1953.

MULDER, D. W. and DALY, D.: Psychiatric symptoms associated with lesions of temporal lobe, J.A.M.A. 150:173, Sept. 20, 1952.

PENFIELD, W.: The Twenty-ninth Maudsley Lecture: The role of the temporal cortex in certain psychical phenomena, J. Ment. Sc. 101:451, July 1955.

PENFIELD, W. and JASPER, H.: Epilepsy and the Functional Anatomy of the Human Brain, Boston, Little, Brown & Company, 1954, pp. 153–4, 438–69, 497–539.

REVITCH, E. and LUZZI, M.: Electroencephalographic survey of a mental hospital (with special reference to temporal lobe abnormalities), Dis. Nerv. System 14:331, Nov. 1953.

RICHARDSON, J. C.: Psychic aspects of cerebral attacks, M. Clin. North America 557, March 1952.

WEIL, A. A.: Ictal depression and anxiety in temporal lobe disorders, Am. J. Psychiat. 113:149, Aug. 1956.

WEINSTEIN, E. A., LINN, L. and KAHN, R. L.: Psychosis during electroshock therapy: Its relation to the theory of shock therapy, Am. J. Psychiat. 109:22, July 1952.

WILLIAMS, D.: Cerebral basis of temperament and personality, Lancet 267:1, July 3, 1954.

——— The structure of emotions reflected in epileptic experiences, Brain 79:29, Part 1, 1956.

PART III

Practical Application
to Clinical Cases

CHAPTER X

Clinical Investigative Approach

As in the analysis of all clinical problems, a systematic detailed history, physical examination and the discriminating use of laboratory and other special investigations is the surest basis for accurate diagnosis. Short cuts can be hazardous. None the less, certain facts in the history and certain abnormal signs on clinical and laboratory examination merit particularly close attention. Thorough search for these clues may prove rewarding. In particular, the following aspects should be carefully assessed.

1. PRESENT ILLNESS

(a) A careful appraisal of the onset of the illness is valuable. An organic psychosis of rapid onset could be due to a vascular accident, an acute infection or a rapidly acting exogenous or endogenous toxin. Conversely, where the onset is gradual, chronic vascular change, neoplasm, degeneration, low grade infection and chronic intoxication are possibilities. The immediate setting in which the illness began should be examined with inquiries made regarding possible exogenous toxins at home or at work, exposure to infection, drugs and the like.

(b) A thorough search for those symptoms we associate with impairment of high level functioning should be made. Patients with organic psychoses tend to display one or more of the following symptoms: defects of comprehension, clouding of consciousness, disorientation, memory impairment, reduction in intellectual efficiency, unusual episodic behaviour including seizures of various sorts, aphasia, defects of judgment, irritability, subtle and even gross changes in personality, emotional apathy and hallucinations, especially visual. Although not necessarily pathognomonic of organic impairment, these symptoms should always be taken as warning signals.

2. PAST HISTORY

A history of long continued medication, drug addiction or self therapy may be important, but such a history is often difficult to elicit. The previous diet should be known in sufficient detail to decide whether nutritional deficiency could be a factor. Particular attention should be paid to the possibility of exposure to toxic materials at work or in the pursuit of hobbies. The psychosis may represent an exacerbation or complication of a chronic illness such as: a malarial infection acquired some years before, meningitis complicating chronic pulmonary tuberculosis or a secondary carcinoma of the brain arising from the lung. A history relatively free of emotional instability in spite of considerable psychological and social stress through the years should immediately suggest the possibility of an organic factor operating in the production of the psychosis. On the other hand, a long history of emotional upsets does not automatically rule out the need to consider a physical element in the present breakdown.

3. FAMILY HISTORY

A family history of any of the following diseases increases the likelihood that the patient may be suffering from the same condition: amaurotic family idiocy, phenylpyruvic oligophrenia, Huntington's chorea, Wilson's disease, Friedreich's ataxia, epilepsy, degenerative vascular disease, porphyria, tuberous sclerosis, Alzheimer's or Pick's disease.

4. FUNCTIONAL INQUIRY

In addition to assessing the mental status for defects in high level cerebral functioning, as was mentioned under "present illness," one should search for the occurrence of other symptoms. Cerebral disease may produce a variety of symptoms including headache, vomiting, defective vision, paraesthesias, paralysis and defects in balancing. A brief routine functional inquiry regarding symptoms concerning the head and neck, lungs, heart, gastro-intestinal tract, genito-urinary system, locomotor system and skin can be amplified by detailed questioning about symptoms suggested by, or elicited in, the assessment of the present illness. For example, if a patient has been suffering from recurring episodes of delirium accompanied by the passage of dark urine one would want full information about abdominal pain, photosensitivity of the skin, and evidence of peripheral neuritis in order to explore the possibility of porphyria.

5. PHYSICAL EXAMINATION

The physical examination begins with the observation of the patient's general physical state, followed by examination of the individual systems. Because the brain is affected in every organic psychosis, localizing neurological signs are often present. Therefore, a thorough neurological examination is of great importance. This is difficult to do in a disturbed patient but by careful observation much can be learned even under such circumstances. It is well to begin with examination of the fundi. If the patient is unco-operative, it may be necessary to administer a sedative and instill 1% homatropine after the pupillary reactions have been noted. The optic discs, vessels and retinae are carefully scrutinized. Auscultation of the eye-balls, cranium and upper portions of the carotid arteries may reveal a bruit indicating the possibility of a vascular abnormality. Then the cranial nerves can be examined, followed by testing of reflexes, observations regarding spontaneous movements, muscle fasciculation, power, tone, co-ordination, gait, tremor and finally the sensory examination. Attention to the other systems and organs: cardiovascular, respiratory, liver, spleen, etc., now follows. A brief glance at the classification of the organic psychoses in chapter II will indicate how wide the scope of this examination must be.

6. LABORATORY INVESTIGATION

Although each test should be done with some specific reason in mind, a certain indispensible minimum, consisting, in part, of the haemoglobin determination, white blood count and examination of a blood smear are necessary because at times the patient's appearance is a poor guide to the haemoglobin content of the blood, and there may be leukopoenia or leukocytosis in the absence of definite clues in the history or physical examination. Furthermore, each patient should have a blood Wasserman test. Similarly, the urine is tested for specific gravity, albumin, sugar, ketones, bile, urobilin, porphyrins and microscopic elements because grave disease may be present without characteristic symptoms.

Good judgment should be exercised in pursuing further laboratory investigation. Although it is wise, where facilities are readily available and the disease process obscure, to search diligently, the indiscriminate use of batteries of tests frequently results in confusion when minor deviations from "normal" are found. The scope of investigation is illustrated by the following outline of procedures which may be helpful in certain instances:

(*a*) A good temperature chart may call for rectal temperatures q.4.h.

(*b*) The haematocrit determination, haemoglobin concentration and smear will indicate the general character of an anaemia. In obscure types, however, the van den Bergh test, reticulocyte count and various tests for agglutinating and haemolysing antibodies may be necessary to clarify the picture. When diffuse collagen disease is suspected, the "L-E" cell test should be done.

(*c*) Chemical blood tests of value include:

> (i) Blood sugars, both fasting and in the glucose tolerance test, which may be helpful in establishing the diagnosis of such conditions as hypoglycaemia, liver disease, anterior pituitary and adrenal disease.

(ii) N.P.N. or blood urea which provide some index of renal function.

(iii) Electrolytes: the concentration of sodium, potassium, calcium, phosphorus, chloride and other electrolytes in the blood, as well as the carbon dioxide combining power, may be altered in dehydration, renal disease, Addison's disease, and other conditions in which diarrhoea or vomiting are present.

(iv) Blood pyruvates—their measurement may be diagnostically valuable in establishing the presence of thiamine deficiency.

(v) Exogenous toxins may be detected in the blood: alcohol, bromides, barbiturates, thiocyanates, lead and sulfonamides are examples.

(d) Urine tests include:

(i) Determinations of renal function, e.g., the two hour Mosenthal, dehydration and diuresis tests.

(ii) Detection of exogenous toxins such as those mentioned in (c) (v) above.

(e) Cerebrospinal fluid examinations, where indicated, may include: gross appearance, pressure, Queckenstedt test, cell count on a fresh specimen, Pandy test for globulin, sugar, chlorides, Wasserman, colloidal gold, total protein determination, smear and culture for bacteria. Certain tests can be made for drugs and other toxins.

(f) The radiological examinations of most value are stereoscopic skull films, which, among other things, may indicate the position of a calcified pineal gland, and air encephalograms. In special cases, ventriculography and angiography provide valuable information. Chest X-ray, gastro-intestinal studies and other investigations may be helpful in certain patients.

(g) The electroencephalogram can be an aid in the diagnosis of a focal lesion, idiopathic epilepsy or diffuse cerebral changes. It is imperative always to consider the electroencephalograph findings, as indeed all laboratory findings, in the light of the total clinical picture.

(h) Where endocrine disease is suspected, basal metabolic rate, radioactive iodine uptake, serum protein-bound iodine, ACTH test and other special tests may be indicated.

(i) Psychological tests particularly designed to demonstrate reduction in intellectual efficiency, memory loss, or other indications of cerebral damage can be most useful diagnostic aids in detecting early cerebral organic change, for example, in such conditions as presenile psychosis, brain tumour, chronic toxic states, cerebral arteriosclerosis.

In brief, the physician may be called upon to use almost every known diagnostic aid to clarify the setting in which an organic psychosis appears.

REFERENCES

General

DEWAN, J. G. and OWEN, T.: Mental illness and the principles of medicine, Canad. M.A.J. 52:349, April 1945. (Several of the cases described in chapters XI, XII and XIII have been reported in this article.)

KAY, D. W. K. and ROTH, M.: Physical accompaniments of mental disorder in old age, Lancet 269:740, Oct. 8, 1955.

ROBERTSON, E. E. and BROWNE, N. L. M.: Review of mental illness in the older age group, Brit. M.J. 2:1076, Nov. 14, 1953.

STOKES, J. F., NABARRO, J. D. N., ROSENHEIM, M. L. and DUNKLEY, E. W.: Physical disease in a mental observation unit, Lancet 267:862, Oct. 23, 1954.

TISSENBAUM, M. J., HARTER, H. M. and FRIEDMAN, A. P.: Organic neurological syndromes diagnosed as functional disorders, J.A.M.A. 147:1519, Dec. 15, 1951.

Others

COHN, J. B., STECKLER, G. A., TAKACS, W. S. and LORENZO, J.: Electroencephalogram and a psychological battery in the diagnosis of organic psychoses, Dis. Nerv. System 13:197, July 1952.

FAUCETT, R. L.: Psychiatric interview as tool of medical diagnosis, J.A.M.A. 162:537, Oct. 6, 1956.

FISHER, J. and GONDA, T. A.: Neurologic techniques and Rorschach test in detecting brain pathology, Arch. Neurol. & Psychiat. 74:117, Aug. 1955.

GOSLING, R. H.: The association of dementia with radiologically demonstrated cerebral atrophy, J. Neurol. Neurosurg. & Psychiat. 18:129, May 1955.

HOPKINS, B. and ROTH, M.: Psychological test performance in patients over sixty: II, Paraphrenia, arteriosclerotic psychosis and acute confusion, J. Ment. Sc. 99:451, July 1953.

PERESE, D. M., KITE, W. C., BEDELL, A. J. and CAMPBELL, E.: Complications following cerebral angiography, Arch. Neurol. & Psychiat. 71:105, Jan. 1954.

ROTH, M. and HOPKINS, B.: Psychological test performance in patients over sixty: I, Senile psychosis and the affective disorders of old age, J. Ment. Sc. 99:439, July 1953.

WEINER, H. and SCHUSTER, D. B.: The electroencephalogram in dementia—some preliminary observations and correlations; Electroencephalog. & Clin. Neurophysiol. 8:479, Aug. 1956.

WEINSTEIN, E. A., KAHN, R. L., SUGARMAN, L. A. and MALITZ, S.: Serial administration of the "amytal test" for brain disease—its diagnostic and prognostic value, Arch. Neurol. & Psychiat. 71:217, Feb. 1954.

ZIEGLER, D. K.: Cerebral atrophy in psychiatric patients, Am. J. Psychiat. 111:454, Dec. 1954.

CHAPTER XI

Diagnostic Orientation

In Parts I and II of this monograph an attempt has been made to discuss briefly and systematically the majority of physical disorders which may include mental symptoms among their manifestations, from a classification we have found helpful. The reader with this background is perhaps in a better position to consider now the organic psychiatric syndromes as they may present to the general physician or to the doctor in the observation ward of a psychiatric hospital, mental hospital or general hospital. It is proposed in this section to focus attention on the strictly clinical, practical level, attempting to convey to the reader our own steps in thinking as patients present themselves. As one's experience increases many of the steps are taken almost automatically without any conscious deliberation. This may be an integral part of the so-called clinical sense so evident in the wise clinician. The student and the clinician new to the field are perhaps well advised to have some systematic, analytical approach, as so frequently the doctor confronted with these psychiatric disorders feels somewhat baffled.

Organic syndromes tend to fall into two groupings: the deliria and the dementias. In addition, there is a third more ill-defined group in which functional mental illness is associated with physical disease involving the brain. These syndromes may be defined or, more correctly, described in the following manner:

Delirium is usually an acute, transient psychiatric disturbance frequently characterized by clouded sensorium, disorientation, irrational thinking, defective judgment, excited, overactive, impulsive behaviour, fearfulness, and illusions and hallucinations, especially visual. It is almost invariably an indication of some physical disorder but on rare occasions one does see delirium associated with severe anxiety or other exhausting emotional disturbance in the absence of physical disease. The patient's memory for recent events may be defective, as a result of the interference with brain functioning. This memory defect is often exaggerated by the bewilderment and preoccupation with disturbing thoughts. Occasionally a delirious state may proceed to mild or severe dementia. It is well to realize that there may be great variability in the degree of severity of delirious states and, furthermore, the symptoms which have been mentioned above need not all be present in the individual case.

By dementia we mean a decrease in mental functioning, usually of a permanent nature, characterized by defects in memory, learning, orientation, abstract thinking, judgment and higher social discrimination. The dementing process may cease with only minimal damage or may proceed to complete deterioration of the personality. Occasionally, when the underlying disturbance is corrected or resolves spontaneously, improvement in mental functioning may be striking.

In addition to delirium and dementia, we should like to consider the group in which functional mental illness is associated with physical disease involving the brain. It is of great practical importance for the clinician to be aware that a mental illness presenting as a functional psychiatric disability (e.g. schizophrenia, depression) is occasionally related to a physical disease process involving the brain. Especially in the early stages there may be no classical signs or symptoms of an organic psychosis but as the condition progresses these findings usually appear. The relationship between the physical disorder and the mental disability may be considered from different points of view:

(*a*) The functional mental illness may be thought of as due to a direct specific effect of the physical disorder on the cells of the central nervous system.

(*b*) Or the physical disease may be considered as an added non-specific stress acting in conjunction with other factors (genetic, personality, psychological) predisposing and contributing to the illness.

(*c*) Or the mental illness may be looked upon as a resultant of both sets of forces mentioned above.

(*d*) Or, of course, there is always the possibility that the two processes may be merely coincidental.

The authors feel that until more is known about physicochemical and psychological mechanisms causing mental illness one should keep an open mind as to this relationship. The case histories in chapter XIV will tend to illustrate these difficulties and it is up to the reader how he relates the psychosis and the physical disorder in each individual case. (Although we have described delirium, dementia and functional mental syndromes as if they were mutually exclusive, it is not uncommon to observe overlapping features of these three groupings in the same patient.)

As was mentioned in the preface, the aim of this monograph is to assist the reader to recognize organic factors in his investigation of mentally ill patients. We would suggest that in proceeding towards a diagnosis the examiner first obtain a brief account of the illness, then make an assessment of the presenting mental picture and carry out a physical examination of the patient. By so doing, he may be able to uncover contributing organic factors quickly and to begin further investigation without delay. Of great practical importance is the fact that the need for prompt physical treatment may be recognized for the first time. Having completed the preliminary survey, one should then be in a position to ask oneself the following questions:

(*a*) Does the patient exhibit features of either delirium or dementia?

If the answer is yes, detailed study of the history and more searching physical investigations should be undertaken, having in mind the factors which most commonly underlie these syndromes, as listed at the beginning of chapters XII and XIII. It it not usually difficult to differentiate between a delirium and a dementia, and some illustrative case reports will be found in the next two chapters. If the answer is no, that is, one finds no evidence of delirium or dementia, the next question is:

(*b*) Is there any indication of a physical disorder which might be disturbing cerebral functioning? If so, the problem is to determine, if possible, the relationship between the physical disorder and the abnormal mental state. Case histories illustrative of the types of problem which may be encountered are presented in chapter XIV. If there is no indication of a physical disorder, the examiner then proceeds in the usual manner of assessment and treatment of a functional mental illness. (It may appear to some that the plan of investigation outlined above is contrary to the principle of a broad approach to the understanding of mental illness in which all factors, psychological, social and physical, are considered as integrated sets of forces; that attempting to investigate the physical aspects at the initial examination fosters diagnosis by exclusion. We feel, however, that the holistic concept can be adhered to, while special attention is given early to possible physical factors in order that time is not lost in dealing with these aspects.)

A word about the case histories in the next three chapters is in order. In the cases we have chosen, the credit for making discerning diagnoses is shared by many doctors with whom we have been associated. These histories have been selected with care from a large number of similar, but from a teaching point of view, less suitable records. The best "teaching case" is often unusually free of confusing features, because in a book of this kind one wishes to show as clearly as possible the part played by the physical disorder in the genesis of the mental illness. We would stress the fact that in some cases the importance of the various physical factors may prove very difficult to assess. For example, many patients who suffer from intoxications due to drugs are mentally unstable and may be taking excessive amounts of alcohol in addition to several potentially intoxicating drugs. In such cases, it may be impossible to sort out the relative importance of the various factors. A demented patient may be thought to be suffering from a presenile cerebral degeneration, but in the absence of a microscopic examination of the brain the diagnosis lacks final confirmation. An alcoholic patient may have a series of grand mal seizures and then become psychotic. In such a case, if a subdural haematoma is then discovered, treated, and the patient recovers, it is very difficult to say whether the psychosis was chiefly due to alcoholism, epilepsy or the subdural haematoma. In other words, even within the area of physical causes, we are frequently confronted with complex factors contributing to the illness. As stated in the preface and referred to briefly in some of the individual cases which follow, this complexity of physical factors must always be considered within the larger framework which includes personality pattern, psychological conflict and social stress.

REFERENCES

BRENNER, C., FRIEDMAN, A. P. and MERRITT, H. H.: Psychiatric syndromes in patients with organic brain disease: 1, Diseases of the basal ganglia, Am. J. Psychiat. 103:733, May 1947.

DEWHURST, K. and PEARSON, J.: Visual hallucinations of the self in organic disease, J. Neurol. Neurosurg. & Psychiat. 18:53, Feb. 1955.

KRAMER, H. C.: Laughing spells in patients, after lobotomy, J. Nerv. & Ment. Dis. 119:517, June 1954.

LASSEN, N. A., MUNCK, O. and TOTTEY, E. R.: Mental function and cerebral oxygen consumption in organic dementia, Arch. Neurol. & Psychiat. 77:126, Feb. 1957.

LEVIN, M.: Perseveration at various levels of complexity, with comments on delirium, Arch. Neurol. & Psychiat. 73:439, April 1955.

MOWBRAY, R. M.: Disorientation for age, J. Ment. Sc. 100:749, July 1954.

NATHANSON, M., BERGMAN, P. S. and GORDON, G. G.: Denial of illness, Arch. Neurol. & Psychiat. 68:380, Sept. 1952.

OLDHAM, A. J.: The effects of temporal lobe lesions on behaviour in paranoid states, J. Ment. Sc. 99:580, July 1953.

PRITCHARD, E. A. B.: The functional symptoms of organic disease of the brain, Lancet 268:363, Feb. 19, 1955.

REINHOLD, M.: Human behaviour reactions to organic cerebral disease, J. Ment. Sc. 99:130, Jan. 1953.

——— Certain disturbances of attention associated with organic cerebral disease, Brain 78:417, Part III, 1955.

SMITH, S.: Organic syndromes presenting as involutional melancholia, Brit. M.J. 2:274, July 31, 1954.

WAGGONER, R. W. and BAGCHI, B. K.: Initial masking of organic brain changes by psychic symptoms, Am. J. Psychiat. 110:904, June 1954.

WEINSTEIN, E. A., KAHN, R. L. and SUGARMAN, L. A.: Phenomenon of reduplication, Arch. Neurol. & Psychiat. 67:808, June 1952.

WEINSTEIN, E. A., KAHN, R. L., MALITZ, S. and ROZANSKI, J.: Delusional reduplication of parts of the body, Brain 77:45, Part I, 1954.

WEINSTEIN, E. A., KAHN, R. L. and SLOTE, W. H.: Withdrawal, inattention and pain asymbolia, Arch. Neurol. & Psychiat. 74:235, Sept. 1955.

ZANGWILL, O. L.: Disorientation for age, J. Ment. Sc. 99:698, Oct. 1953.

CHAPTER XII

Delirium

Generally speaking there is no specific mental picture for each cause of delirium. Investigation requires a knowledge of the chief physical and chemical aetiological factors responsible for delirious states. We would suggest the following classification:

1. Intoxications
2. Metabolic disorders
3. Infections
4. Cardiovascular disorders
5. Trauma
6. Epilepsy
7. Other settings for delirium

The following cases illustrate some of the salient features of these conditions.

1. INTOXICATIONS

Case 1

The patient, a twenty-six year old woman, was transferred from a general hospital to a psychiatric hospital because of the development of a mental illness. On admission she was drowsy, her remarks were irrelevant and incoherent, and she appeared hallucinated and disoriented. This presenting picture is typical of an organic mental illness of the delirious type. About five weeks previously she had injured her back when thrown from a horse. She continued to complain of soreness of the back and was admitted to a general hospital for investigation. Because she appeared to be very nervous and restless, a bromide mixture was prescribed, each dose containing gr. xxv, to be taken three times a day. After three weeks of this medication, her mental state had reached the point described above, and she could no longer be managed in a general hospital.

Thus, on the basis of the presenting picture and the history, it appeared obvious that the illness not only was a toxic delirious state but in all probability was due to the bromide. Accordingly, the amount of bromide in the blood was measured on the second hospital day and found to be 400 mg. per 100 ml. No medication was given apart from the occasional administration of nembutal. Within a week she had definitely improved, having become less confused and disoriented. By the twelfth hospital day she appeared completely recovered, was clear in her thinking and displayed insight into her condition. This improvement coincided closely with a fall in the blood bromide which was 235 mg. per 100 ml. on the eighth day in hospital and 80 mg. per 100 ml. on the eighteenth day.

As more information was obtained, it was found that this woman had always been an immature individual who overreacted emotionally to difficult situations. It was felt that she was reacting excessively to the accident and the discomfort of her injury. Because of this the sedative was prescribed. As is so often the case when sedatives are employed in emotionally upset individuals, the physician may deal with the increasingly disturbed state by continuing the sedative, not realizing that the picture has now shifted to one that is predominantly organic.

Case 2

The patient, aged fifty-five, was admitted to a general hospital because she was extremely apprehensive, suspicious and heard voices and sounds that terrified her. This mental picture in itself could be indicative of either a functional mental illness such as an acute paranoid state or an organic psychosis. The steps in arriving at a diagnosis were as follows:

(a) As the patient was observed further it was noted that she was unable to enunciate clearly and had visual hallucinations, stating that she could see devils. These points favoured the possibility of an organic state, and the paranoid trends, for example fear that she was being poisoned and accusing the nurse that she was filling her with electricity, are compatible with an organic psychiatric syndrome. However, there were no positive findings on examination with the exception of a two-plus albuminuria.

(b) At this stage the only relevant history obtainable was the statement by the referring physician that she had consulted him twelve days previously and he had found her blood pressure to be 250/140 mm. Hg. He considered her mental illness to be a manifestation of hypertensive encephalopathy but the hospital physicians were unable to find evidence of this condition. For example, the husband stated that she had had no severe headaches or vomiting. The admission blood pressure was only 140/88 mm. Hg and the optic fundi were free of haemorrhages or exudates.

(c) Further information from the husband gave the first leads pointing to the organic nature of the illness and to the causative factor. He stated that she had always been a happy, stable person. Twelve days before admission she felt dizzy, and her physician on finding the blood pressure to be elevated, prescribed some pills; ten days later she had become confused, tearful and was unable to speak clearly; medication was discontinued but her mental state worsened. The fact that she had always had good mental health until two days before admission, followed by a rapidly deteriorating mental state with certain delirious features coincident with some form of medication, raised the possibility of a drug intoxication.

(d) Because her general practitioner could not be reached, the prescription was traced to the druggist, and it was learned that the patient had been taking sodium thiocyanate grains iii, four times a day. As it is known that intoxications due to thiocyanate occur not infrequently it seemed logical to check the serum level and this was found to be 20 mg. per 100 ml. (A serum level above 12 is considered to be hazardous.) This finding, plus a negative test for bromide in the serum and only a moderate elevation of non-protein nitrogen, made the diagnosis of thiocyanate intoxication probable. The diagnosis was considered to be confirmed by improvement in the mental state coincident with a falling level of thiocyanate in serum and cerebrospinal fluid.

Seven years later this patient was well and carrying on with her housework. The blood pressure continued to be elevated.

Case 3

The patient, aged thirty-nine, was known to have been "a rather heavy drinker" for a number of years. A few weeks before admission to hospital he began to drink more heavily and was worrying greatly over his wife's health. His condition became complicated by the development of hallucinations and a fearful state. The patient's father managed to persuade him to come to hospital voluntarily. He was obviously quite disturbed and ran out of the hospital. Some hours later the police reported that they had taken him into custody, as he was observed attempting to throw himself in front of motor cars. He told the police that he heard people telling him that his father had died. In the police station he thrust his right hand through a pane of glass, sustaining a laceration of the hand and wrist. He was taken to a general hospital where the lacerations were sutured. A small abrasion on the forehead was noted. As the patient continued to be actively hallucinating and frightened, he was transferred to a psychiatric hospital.

On admission he was very agitated, at times talking rationally at other times laughing inappropriately. On occasion it was obvious that he was hallucinating and would shout, "Look out, they're looking in the window." The admission physical examination, including a detailed neurological examination, disclosed a blood pressure of 180/110 mm. Hg but otherwise was completely negative. The day following admission his behaviour was, for the most part, quiet and co-operative, although at times it was apparent that he was hallucinating. On one occasion he stated that he could hear his wife's voice out in the hall, although she was not in the hospital at the time. On another occasion he expressed concern that his coffee had been poisoned. Later in the day the nurse reported that he appeared slightly depressed; he slept fitfully that night with the aid of sedatives. At 4:15 A.M. he jumped impulsively out of bed and attempted to attack the attendant, shouting, "There was a collection taken up yesterday and you are keeping my share." This outburst subsided quickly and he returned to bed. At 7 A.M. the nurse was unable to arouse him for the day. On examination he was stuporous, his breathing was stertorous and there was a decided change in neurological findings. The right pupil was dilated and fixed, the left small and fixed; the discs were moderately choked. The left arm and leg were spastic and Babinski reflexes were present bilaterally. The patient moved the right arm much more than the left.

It was considered that there was a strong possibility of an intracranial haemorrhage, and after consultation with a neurosurgeon, the patient was transferred immediately to a general hospital. The neurological findings were confirmed and a lumbar puncture revealed the cerebrospinal fluid to be slightly tinged with blood. It appeared obvious that the condition demanded craniotomy at once. At operation, a very large subdural haematoma was found, covering the entire right cerebral hemisphere, with the brain pushed about one inch away from the dura. A bleeding vessel was found on the surface of the brain in the parietal region.

The following day he was much improved. He was conscious, answered simple questions appropriately, but at times his conversation was irrational. Both pupils reacted promptly to light. His recovery was delayed by the presence of a small abscess deep to the incision in the scalp. Following evacuation of the abscess, the patient rapidly recovered, and five weeks after admission to the general hospital, he was discharged. At that time there were no longer any evidences of hallucinations, thought disorder or unusual behaviour.

This case illustrates a number of interesting points:

(a) It is rather typical of acute hallucinosis associated with excessive intake of alcohol over a prolonged period.

(b) This type of florid picture makes one suspect that the alcohol is not only toxic to the central nervous system but has released abnormal personality trends. Following discharge of the patient from hospital, we were able to obtain reliable information about his previous personality. He was described as always being a very jealous man, suspicious of any person who even spoke to his wife and very angry with his wife if she was out of the house, even if she only went to the store. He had had few interests or recreations and had no really close friends.

(c) A diagnosis of alcoholic intoxication may lead one to ignore the possibility of some other contributing or complicating factor, for example, an infection such as meningitis or pneumonia, or, as in this case, a subdural haematoma. Not infrequently, such a complication leads to sudden deterioration in the patient's physical state, necessitating quick decision as to diagnosis and treatment.

(d) The case also illustrates the difficulty of obtaining a history of any significant head injury in some cases of subdural haematoma. The abrasion on the forehead noted on admission was the only indication of head injury that was obtained.

Case 4

This man, aged sixty-one, was admitted to a general hospital in a semicomatose condition, hallucinated, fearful, very restless and talking incoherently. He became rapidly more disturbed, and would hide behind chairs and the bed saying that he saw animals in the room. Because it was felt that the patient was unmanageable in the general hospital, no extensive investigations were initiated and he was transferred to a psychiatric hospital as a case of functional mental illness.

There were three major leads in this case:

(*a*) The history obtained from the wife indicated that this man had always been a very stable person, but in the past four months his general health deteriorated in that he complained of dizziness, loss of appetite, headaches and tiring easily. For the two weeks before admission to hospital, he had urinary frequency both day and night, more severe headaches, vomiting and difficulty in remembering things. This history of an emotionally stable person rather abruptly developing an illness with certain physical features such as severe headaches, vomiting and memory dysfunction should be a warning to the examiner that physical factors may be playing important roles.

(*b*) The story of visual hallucinations and fear in the general hospital lend further weight to this likelihood. These symptoms plus the memory disorder are characteristic of the delirious type of organic psychosis.

(*c*) With the exception of Cheyne-Stokes respirations, physical findings were of little aid. The third major clue was the urinary findings, which consisted of a specific gravity of 1.010, one plus albumin and occasional granular and cellular casts and white blood cells. These findings might have been ignored as of no special significance had not the history and the mental picture alerted the examiner to be on the watch for any lead as to a toxic factor. On the chance that this man might be suffering from uraemia, a blood non-protein nitrogen was ordered and the result the day after admission was 171 mg. per 100 ml. Three days later, the non-protein nitrogen was 119 mg. per 100 ml. with a concurrent improvement in his mental state. He was becoming less confused, quieter and talking more rationally. By the fifth hospital day there were no mental symptoms except inability to remember events which had occurred during the acute stage of the illness. This memory defect is typical of delirious states. Two days later he was quite clear in his thinking, pleasant, co-operative and aware of his surroundings. Non-protein nitrogen, by this time, was 40 mg. per 100 ml. Subsequent tests revealed some impairment of renal function and it was felt that the uraemic episode was due to an exacerbation of either chronic glomerulonephritis or chronic pyelonephritis.

2. METABOLIC DISORDERS

Case 5*

While this case presented no major difficulty in the recognition of the organic nature of the illness, it is being quoted because it illustrates rather well the interrelationship of the biochemical and the mental abnormalities. Furthermore, it points up the complexities and difficulties a physician frequently encounters in attempting to establish the specific underlying disorder.

The patient was a fifty-six year old office worker who had always been considered a stable person. His health had been good until March 8, 1953, when he became irritable and began to tire easily. Because of these continuing symptoms the family doctor was called. The doctor, attributing these symptoms to overwork and nervous exhaustion, prescribed bromide and phenobarbital medication. On March 16, the patient was feverish and perspiring profusely. The next day he became drowsy; relatives described his eyes as glazed and they noticed a dusky red flush on his face. During March 19 and 20, he passed about 10 or 12 soft, brown stools involuntarily. This was the only time diarrhoea occurred. He ate and drank little during these days of acute illness. On March 22 he was sweating, feverish and sleeping long periods, but if roused was

*This case was described in an article by W. B. Spaulding, W. A. Oille, and A. G. Gornall, Mineralocorticoid-like disturbance associated with adrenal metastases from a bronchogenic carcinoma, Ann. Int. Med. 42:444, Feb. 1955. Diagram reproduced by kind permission of the Editor.

alert enough to recognize and talk to relatives. It was obvious to the attending physician that this was an acute physical disorder requiring investigation and treatment in hospital.

Physical examination on admission to hospital on March 23, 1953, showed him to be obese (usual weight 218 lbs.) very drowsy and severely dehydrated. His face was flushed and cyanotic. His blood pressure was 130/70 mm. Hg. He exhibited some signs of delirium in that he was disoriented as to time and place but was able to recognize his wife, a friend and his own doctor.

The admission urine specimen contained two plus sugar and the fasting blood sugar on the following day was 388 mg. per 100 ml. The next day, March 25, the fasting blood sugar was 335 mg. and the carbon dioxide combining power 97 vol. per 100 ml. On March 26, blood sugar was 375 mg., carbon dioxide combining power 114 vol., serum potassium 10 mg., chloride (as NaC1) 432 mg. and sodium 336 mg. per 100 ml. The blood pH was 7.7 on March 27. This combination of hypopotassemia, hypochloremia and alkalosis is rarely seen apart from the state of overactivity of the adrenal cortex. Accordingly, adrenocortical function was investigated as follows: Absolute eosinophil counts on March 27 and 29 were 11 and 44 per c. mm. respectively. Urinary 17-keto-steroids were found to be within normal limits but urinary corticoids were over 8 mg. per 24 hours which is considered about four times the normal excretion for a man of this age by the particular method which was employed. These findings were compatible with overactivity of the adrenal cortex.

The accompanying figure shows the biochemical state and treatment throughout the period in hospital. The patient's mental state appeared to correlate with the biochemical disturbance. On March 24 he said there were mice running around in his bed and trains passing by the window of his room (on the fourth floor). He referred to non-existent pictures on the wall. It rained on March 25 and he reported that water was coming from the hoses of firemen. He claimed

HYPERADRENALCORTICISM

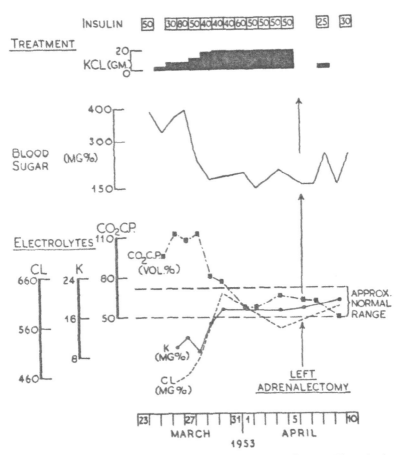

to see friends in the room when none were there. His mind cleared somewhat by March 26, but although he knew the month, his family doctor's name and the fact that he had a cholecystectomy three years previously, he could not remember events in the immediate past. From this time until April 1 he was drowsy and somewhat confused about the surroundings, visitors and the time of day. After the electrolyte upset had been corrected (see figure) his mental state improved and remained clear.

In view of the above biochemical findings plus evidence of an adrenal tumour by intravenous pyelography a laparotomy was performed. An adrenal tumour was removed. The patient only survived a few days postoperatively. Autopsy revealed this tumour to be a metastatic growth secondary to a bronchogenic carcinoma. The exact basis of his adrenal cortical hyperfunction remained obscure. However, it seemed apparent that the disturbed mental state was closely related to the biochemical abnormality.

Case 6

While the following case presented no serious difficulty in diagnosis, it is rather a good example of a delirious state related to hyperfunction of the thyroid gland.

On admission to a psychiatric hospital, this patient, aged thirty-seven, was excited, hallucinated and in extreme fear. He was very restless, attempted to jump out of bed, and felt that patients and staff were trying to shoot him. He refused food, fearing poison. He was thin, his skin was moist, the pulse rapid (120); examination of the eyes revealed exophthalmos and pronounced lid lag. There was much vasodilatation, a fine generalized tremor, and a diffusely enlarged and nodular thyroid. The heart was regular with a short, sharp, first sound.

The previous history of this man indicated that he had always been a stable individual, pleasant and a good mixer. He had had a steady work record. During the past two years he had been losing weight, tiring easily and perspiring a good deal. A physician examined him, made a diagnosis of hyperthyroidism and admitted him to a general hospital. After a few days he became excited and apprehensive, feared poisoning and made attempts to escape from the hospital. It was then that he was transferred to a psychiatric hospital. He was given Lugol's solution, 10 minims twice a day, in preparation for thyroidectomy and in three days he had become quiet, there was no apprehension, no hallucinations or delusions and he was sleeping well without sedatives. He was quite lucid, gave a clear history and had complete insight into his condition. He was operated on after ten days of preoperative Lugol's solution and made a good recovery. His mental state was quite satisfactory when re-examined two years later.

3. INFECTION

In recent years, owing to the widespread use of antibiotics, most acute infections are being treated early and effectively with the result that associated deliria are becoming less frequent. The following case was encountered before the introduction of antibiotics. It illustrates the difficulties which can still arise in diagnosing such an illness.

Case 7

This man, aged fifty-two, was admitted to a psychiatric hospital in a very excited, resistive condition. He tossed about violently, and his conversation was incoherent. Even with heavy sedation he had very little rest. Investigation of the history indicated that he had always been a quiet, well-adjusted man, who held a responsible position as an engineer with a construction company. He was working until the day before admission, when he came home at 2 P.M. complaining of a violent headache. He lay down and slept until 6 P.M. At 9 P.M. he became restless, talked incoherently and vomited. The family physician was called and the patient's temperature was 101° F. After being given a sedative hypodermically, he slept until 3 A.M. the next morning. Upon awakening, he became progressively more restless and disturbed; he frequently held his head, and would get up on his hands and knees with his head down. He was becoming so uncontrollable that it was necessary to admit him to hospital.

Physical examination was difficult to perform, but was essentially negative. The temperature was only 99.2° F., an elevation often encountered in overactive, anxious and disturbed patients. Although the admitting physician recognized that the patient was delirious, he did not consider that there was any immediate need to carry out special investigations. In spite of sedation, the patient remained mentally disturbed. By the following day the physical findings had altered: the right pupil was now slightly larger than the left and reacted sluggishly to light; blood pressure had risen to 190/120 mm. Hg and stiffness of the neck was pronounced; the temperature was 100° F.; the pulse varied from 64 to 120; the white blood count was 5,900 per cu. mm. As a result of consultations with an internist and a neurosurgeon, the possibility of a subarachnoid haemorrhage was considered and a lumbar puncture was therefore done. Surprisingly, the cerebrospinal fluid was turbid and no blood was present. Pus cells were abundant and gram-negative diplococci were present. (These were later identified by culture as meningococci.) The patient was at once transferred to an isolation hospital where he died four days later in spite of intensive chemotherapy with sulfonamides.

This case of meningitis is unusual because physical abnormalities were delayed in appearance, the temperature was only moderately elevated, and the white blood count was normal. However, the history of sudden onset of severe headache and delirium should have immediately raised the question of serious intracranial disease necessitating prompt, special investigation.

4. CARDIOVASCULAR DISORDER

Case 8

The main reason for presenting this case is to show how cardiac dysfunction may interfere with cerebral function and give rise to a mental disturbance, in this case a delirium.

The patient was a fifty-eight year old man who had been a highly successful executive without any history of a previous psychiatric disorder. He had enjoyed good physical health until four years before admission, when he was found to be diabetic and was treated with 40 units of protamine zinc insulin daily. Three months prior to this admission, he suffered from a moderately severe attack of myocardial infarction for which he was treated in hospital for five weeks, subsequently making an uneventful recovery.

Two days before admission he had a second myocardial infarction. During the next few days he was dangerously ill with signs of cardiac failure and shock.

He was readmitted, and five days later there was mental clouding, disorientation and paranoidal thinking. He accused the staff of the hospital of trying to kill him "by experimenting on me and injecting air into my veins." He ripped several oxygen tents, struggled violently to get out of bed, fought with the nursing staff, and despite heavy sedation including H.M.C.'s every two hours, he remained unmanageable.

It was necessary to transfer him to a psychiatric hospital at 3:30 A.M. on the seventh hospital day. On admission to the psychiatric hospital, he was found to be in cardiac failure, with cyanosis, bilateral basal rales and enlargement of the liver. His blood pressure was 100/78 mm. Hg, there was a gallop rhythm and a heart rate of 120 per minute. He was orthopnoeic, breathing at 30 respirations per minute.

The admitting physician was faced, in this case, with an obvious, serious, delirious state and a coexisting, critical, cardiac condition. While he could not discount the possibility that the psychological impact of the knowledge of a serious heart condition on the patient could have contributed to the delirious state, the physician felt that in view of the marked cardiac failure, with gallop rhythm and tachycardia, most likely the cerebral circulation would be deficient. He considered the possibility of hypoglycaemic encephalopathy, but at no time during the illness was the blood sugar found to be below normal. Therefore, in co-operation with the cardiac and psychiatric consultants, he instituted treatment directed towards both the circulatory and cerebral disorders. At this time, the patient was still very disturbed and on one occasion jumped out of bed, grabbed a chair and ran down the hall shouting, "Help, murder!" He was then given 25 mg. of chlorpromazine intravenously and 25 mg. intramuscularly. In addition, he received intravenous digoxin, 2 ml. of thiomerin and oxygen by mask. Chlorpromazine was administered intramuscularly repeatedly. By the following day the patient was less disturbed but still exhibited paranoid thinking. The gallop rhythm had disappeared. His mental and physical state continued to improve in the next few days and on the fourth day, he was correctly orientated, had a good memory and a clear sensorium, and recognized that his ideas and behaviour had been part of an illness. The signs of cardiac failure had disappeared.

5. TRAUMA

Delirious, confused states may follow head injury. The mental state is not especially different from delirious states due to other causes. It is only rarely that the causative factor of trauma is overlooked. Often there is evidence of injury to the head which together with a history of an accident or involvement in a fight gives a clue to the aetiology. Occasionally the fact that the patient has been drinking may lead to the examiner concluding that the mental state is solely due to the alcoholic intoxication whereas head injury may have occurred as a result of an accident or involvement in a fight.

In our experience the cause of delirium in such cases has usually been obvious and we have not considered it necessary to describe a case.

6. EPILEPSY

Case 9

This man, aged forty-five, was brought by the police to the Emergency department of a general hospital. He had been found by the police in an empty garage beating his head against the wall and talking excitedly. His face was badly bruised and bleeding, evidently as a result of the self-injury.

It was difficult to examine him in the Emergency department because he was obviously reacting to hallucinations, shouting out that the Communists were going to kill him; that he had seen a skeleton hanging up on a neighbour's house; that he had seen a man sawing up another man. He was extremely terrified and so disturbed that admission to a mental hospital had to be arranged immediately.

Following admission to the mental hospital, he continued in a disturbed state, frequently knelt and prayed, cried, and clapped his hands together manneristically. He was impulsive and on one occasion smashed his fist through a window. Under heavy sedation it was possible to examine him physically. There were no signs of skull defects and although the possibility of a subdural haematoma was kept in mind, all neurological findings were normal. The presenting clinical picture could be described as a delirium and yet in keeping with an acute manic or schizophrenic illness. The wife was interviewed both at the Emergency department and following the patient's admission to the mental hospital. She stated that the patient had been subject to seizures off and on since childhood and that following a drinking bout, he had had a series of ten convulsions over a period of forty-eight hours preceding his discovery by the police. This information plus the statement by the wife that there had been no noticeable change in personality over the years raised the likelihood that this illness was of the nature of a post-epileptic furor or delirium.

For the next two to three days in hospital he continued to be disturbed. There were intervals of quiet but most of the time he appeared to be responding to visual and auditory hallucinations. He would mutter his prayers unceasingly. He said that he had visions of going up to Heaven and that a battle ensued between God and the Devil. On chlorpromazine his disturbed state subsided, the hallucinations disappeared, and he became pleasant, co-operative and clear in his thinking. It is interesting to note that the wife described a similar acute illness eighteen months previously following a series of seizures. The delirious state persisted for four days on that occasion.

Although the patient was quite recovered from his disturbed state he was kept in hospital in order to obtain a more detailed history and to carry out further investigations. The points in his history of significance are as follows. When he was a small boy he is said to have fallen off a hayrick on his head. Whether this story of a head injury is of significance or not, he had seizures from that time on. The patient stated that preceding the fits he had a feeling of dizziness followed by an unpleasant odour and a vague feeling of abdominal discomfort. These prodromal symptoms were not always followed by a seizure. In the seizures, his wife had observed him to lose consciousness, froth at the mouth, pass through a tonic and clonic phase followed by apnoea, then stertorous breathing and confusion giving place to sleep; in other words a rather typical grand mal seizure. The fits had occurred three or four times a year but in recent years they had become more frequent. Detailed neurological examination and skull films were normal but the electroencephalogram revealed slow waves arising in the right temporal lobe. This finding was considered to be in keeping with an epileptic focus in this part of the brain.

Since the patient had never had adequate anticonvulsant therapy he was placed on an appropriate regimen of drugs. One year later he was well, working steadily and free of seizures.

7. OTHER SETTINGS FOR DELIRIUM

It is well to keep in mind that symptoms of a delirious nature are not infrequently observed in acute manic states, in agitated depressions and elderly individuals especially following surgical procedures such as the removal of cataracts. (In this connection it might be well to mention that fever may occur in some mental illnesses in the absence of any detectable cause such as an infection. This observation applies particularly to acute manic illnesses, catatonic schizophrenics and excited patients in general. Thus in delirious states the presence of a fever does not necessarily mean that there is an infectious disorder present.)

REFERENCES

GILLIES, H.: Acute delirious states, Brit. M.J. 1:623, March 17, 1956.

JARVIE, H. F. and HOOD, M. C.: Acute delirious mania, Am. J. Psychiat. 108:758, April 1952.

CHAPTER XIII

Dementia

We offer the following simple, clinical classification as a guide to the consideration of diagnosis within this group:

1. Primary degeneration of the brain
2. Space-occupying lesions
3. Infections
4. Deficiency states
5. Cardiovascular disorders
6. Anoxia
7. Metabolic disorders
8. Trauma and other settings for dementia

1. PRIMARY DEGENERATION OF THE BRAIN

Case 10

The following case illustrates, in rather typical fashion, the history and findings which may be encountered in a primary cerebral degeneration, namely Alzheimer's disease. The patient, at the time of her admission to hospital, was aged fifty-nine. There was no history of mental illness in the family, and her health, until recent years, had been good. She had been an intelligent girl, had obtained her senior matriculation in a private school, was active socially and had a special interest in oil-painting and needlework. In her early adult life she is stated to have taken alcohol excessively, but there is no subsequent history of excessive intake.

Six years before admission to hospital, her husband died and her only son was killed while on military service. She was very shocked by these deaths and from that time her general physical health seemed to deteriorate gradually. One year before admission it became obvious that her memory was failing; for example, she would forget where she left her purse and would repeat herself. At times she became confused, not knowing where she was or where she was going. Later, she refused to get out of bed or help herself in any way. She became completely disoriented, exhibited a nominal aphasia and had to be certified to a mental hospital.

In hospital, her mental condition continued to deteriorate slowly, to the point that memory was defective for remote as well as recent events. Her conversation was disconnected and difficult to follow; at times she became quite excited. She was oblivious to her personal appearance. Her appetite diminished, there was a gradual loss of weight and she finally died three years following admission, of a terminal bronchopneumonia.

The clinical diagnosis on admission and throughout the stay in hospital was presenile psychosis—Alzheimer's disease.

At autopsy, the brain was found to be small, weighing only 1,055 grams. There was severe cortical atrophy of the frontal and parietal lobes, much more marked on the left side. There was moderate internal hydrocephalus, chiefly involving the left lateral ventricle. The arteries of the brain were almost completely free of atheromatous change. Microscopically, there was a severe loss of nerve cells and myelin sheaths in the cortex and white matter of the frontal lobes. In this region there were Alzheimer tangles, mild gliosis and senile plaques. The pathological diagnosis was Alzheimer's disease.

(We are indebted to Prof. E. A. Linell for providing the report of the autopsy.)

2. SPACE-OCCUPYING LESIONS

Case 11

This fifty-three year old married woman was admitted to a psychiatric hospital by a psychiatrist who stated on the certificate that she was "apathetic, disinterested, mildly depressed, refuses to walk although fracture of femur has healed well;

dominating her family by this disability." Nine months previous to admission, the patient slipped and fell, sustaining a fracture of the right hip. She was taken to a general hospital where the hip was nailed and she was discharged home in one month's time. The fracture was considered completely healed within five months and the doctor was well satisfied with the result. However, the patient remained in bed seeming unable to walk. About three months before admission to the psychiatric hospital she became despondent and "fed up" and was disinclined to enter into conversation. She lost interest in her appearance, neglecting to wash and dress herself and occasionally even to feed herself. As she was showing no improvement and becoming increasingly more of a problem for the family to cope with, it was decided to admit her to a psychiatric hospital.

The description of the psychiatrist who first saw the patient, and the account of the family, strongly suggested the possibility of a depressive reaction. However, the hospital physician noted, within a matter of hours following admission, that there were certain features of the mental status which raised the question of an organic factor. He was especially impressed by the incorrectness of some of her answers and the presence of some mental confusion. Furthermore, there was even a definite memory loss with confabulation. These unexpected findings alerted him to the possibility of organic mental illness, thereby stimulating him to search more carefully than usual for corroborative evidence in the history. It also led to a more detailed and meticulous assessment of the mental status and investigation for neurological abnormalities.

It was learned from the family that the patient had always had good health until five years before, when, at the age of forty-eight, she suddenly had a series of "fits" which resulted in her admission to a general hospital. The hospital record indicated that, on the day of admission, she had had a series of six or seven convulsions of grand mal type. Between the convulsions she was either unconscious or confused. A few hours later she was aware of her surroundings though drowsy. The next day she was clear in her thinking and neurological examination was negative. A lumbar puncture was done but the cerebrospinal fluid was negative in very respect. All laboratory findings, including an air encephalogram, were normal. The final diagnosis on discharge was epilepsy, the treatment recommended being small doses of anticonvulsant drugs. She continued with anticonvulsant medication, had about six grand mal seizures in the next two years and none in the three years previous to her admission to the psychiatric hospital.

Further careful assessment of the mental status confirmed the initial indication of memory loss and confabulation, and in addition, there was evidence of defective orientation. When asked the date, the patient knew what month it was but not the day nor was she sure of the year. She was unaware of what hospital she was in and misidentified the staff and relatives. These defects in mental functioning were sufficiently definite to preclude the need of special psychological investigations.

Although the fundi were normal and the cranial nerves intact, the deep reflexes on the right side were increased and there was a Babinski response on testing the right plantar reflex. These positive neurological findings confirmed the likelihood of a cerebral lesion which had first been suspected because of the organic mental symptoms.

Skull X-rays, electroencephalography and air studies were therefore done. The skull X-rays failed to reveal any abnormality and the air encephalogram was not successful in demonstrating the ventricular system. The report of the electroencephalographer was: "There is a large amount of slow waves in this electroencephalogram, mainly in two ranges of frequency: 2 to 3 per second waves are seen on the left side especially in the temporal lobe, whereas 6 to 7 per second waves are to be found throughout the cortex randomly as well as bilaterally synchronous. The left temporal electrode also shows considerable intermittent 5 per second activity. Impression: Diffuse brain damage with probability of a gross lesion deep in the left temporal area."

In order to localize the lesion a ventriculogram was done. The report of the radiologist may be summarized as follows: "The septum pellucidum measures five mm. to the right of the midline. Both frontal horns are deformed, the defect being greater on the left side than on the right. The shadow of the corpus callosum anteriorly is increased and the roofs of the bodies of the lateral ventricles are separated further than normal. There is very suggestive evidence of an amorphous collection of calcium just anterior to the left frontal horn. The third ventricle, aqueduct and fourth ventricle are not filled (this finding probably explains the unsuccessful air encephalogram). There is air in the callosal cistern and it is displaced forward indicating increase in the size of the corpus callosum." It was the opinion of the radiologist that these findings indicated a diffuse, infiltrating tumour in the corpus callosum extending posteriorly from the frontal horn well into the bodies of the lateral ventricles.

A needle biopsy of the tumour was done, the tissue proving to be a cellular astrocytoma infiltrating normal brain tissue. It was considered that the tumour was inoperable.

The patient's mental and physical state gradually deteriorated and she died a few months later.

Case 12

This man, aged forty-one, was admitted to a psychiatric hospital on a magistrate's warrant. His wife said that his manner had been peculiar for the past year and that he had finally struck her. On the advice of the family physician it was decided that a charge of assault must be laid.

On admission he appeared confused, was unsteady and acted as if intoxicated. His memory for recent events was poor. He was untidy and would urinate on the floor. At times he complained of severe headaches, sudden in onset and of short duration. As these symptoms were strongly suggestive of organic disease of the brain, the attending physician was especially interested in learning of the onset of the mental illness with reference to previous personality and other symptoms indicative of cerebral disease. His wife stated that he had always been a well-adjusted, cheerful person who had many friends. He had worked as a florist's assistant for some years until fourteen months previously when he had a difference of opinion with his employer regarding overtime, the disagreement resulting in his discharge from the job. One wonders if this dispute with his employer, which was foreign to his usual behaviour, might not indeed have been the first sign of the developing mental illness. He was unable to obtain work quickly, appeared despondent and would sit by himself for long periods. His behaviour frequently would be facetious, he would laugh for no apparent reason and when questioned would make irrelevant remarks. Six months previous to admission, it was noticed by the patient's family that he had a squint and the patient complained of seeing double. His mental symptoms became more pronounced, he appeared sullen and preoccupied, sitting staring into space for long periods. In the four months previous to admission he often cried out, "my head, my head", and then would laugh. The last few weeks before coming into hospital the patient stated that he expected the Devil daily at 3 P.M. He thought people were outside the window. He complained of crawling feelings up the back of his head and misidentified relatives. It was only when he struck his wife that she finally consulted a physician and this led to his admission to hospital.

The significant findings were as follows: internal strabismus of the right eye; both pupils reacted to light but the right was sluggish; a questionable weakness of the right hand grip; a tendency to fall to the right side; marked papilloedema bilaterally. All other findings were negative except for a one-plus sugar reaction in the urine.

The history and mental and physical findings were in keeping with a space-occupying lesion. At operation, a large meningioma (the size of an orange and weighing 105 grams) was present in the midline, growing from the longitudinal sinus and falx and impinging on both frontal lobes. The patient did not survive the operation.

Meningioma is the most favourable type of brain tumour to remove. An early careful examination might have indicated the organic lesion. In reviewing the case it would seem that there was a wealth of signs suggesting the likelihood of an underlying organic process involving the brain: striking personality changes a year prior to admission in a man of previous stable personality; six months before admission, strabismus and double vision; complaints of sudden, severe headaches of short duration; memory defect for recent events associated with a generally confused mental state with disorientation and deterioration of finer sensibilities and personal habits; and finally the neurological findings, particularly the advanced papilloedema.

Case 13

This twenty-eight year old labourer was admitted to a mental hospital with a diagnosis of schizophrenia. The medical certificates described the patient as apathetic, slovenly, disoriented and confused. The patient was unable to give a coherent history. His wife stated that he had been ill for over three years: the first symptoms were loss of appetite, a desire to sleep continually and a gradual decrease in interest in his work and his home. At times he had seemed mentally normal but at other times he complained that he could not remember things from one hour to the next and occasionally would come home from work at night and a short while later ask his wife to pack his lunch because he had to go to work. Sometimes he did not know where he was. He could be heard talking to himself at night and on one occasion claimed he had overheard a telephone conversation in which a man threatened to kill the patient's wife.

Examination in hospital disclosed a much retarded man who did not initiate conversation and mistakenly thought his doctor was the father of one of his friends. At times, he was incontinent of urine and faeces and would soil the floor. Within the first month in the mental hospital his condition deteriorated with the development of a stuporous state. The depth of this stupor and the fact that the patient failed to show any of the signs of mental functioning that one expects to see, at times, in the stupor of a catatonic schizophrenic raised the very serious question as to whether an organic factor might be involved. This possibility was further strengthened when an examination of the spinal fluid revealed a protein of 85 mg. per 100 ml. and a paretic type of gold curve. The Wasserman reaction, however, was normal. He was transferred to a general hospital for further investigation.

On admission to the general hospital, he was stuporous, mute and helpless. The following significant findings were obtained on physical examination: unequal pupils; right facial weakness; hyperactive tendon reflexes in the right leg; there was no papilloedema; blood pressure was 90/70 mm. Hg. The first night following admission, the patient became deeply comatose with stertorous breathing and the plantar responses were now bilaterally extensor. The most likely diagnosis was space-occupying lesion. A ventriculogram revealed the presence of a lesion obstructing both foramina of Monro; the lateral ventricles were grossly enlarged and the septum pellucidum was shifted 7 mm. to the right. In spite of several attempts, it was impossible to inject air into the third ventricle. It was the radiologist's opinion that the lesion was an infiltrating one, probably involving the septum pellucidum and the splenium of the corpus callosum. The patient's physical condition was deteriorating rapidly and an exploratory operation was decided upon. The right anterior horn was entered and the interventricular septum could be seen bulging into it. A large opening was made in the septum. Pale, gelatinous, tumour tissue could be seen below the ependymal lining of the floors of the lateral ventricles and surrounding the foramina of Monro. It was decided that the tumour was inoperable. The patient died sixteen days after the operation.

At autopsy, a soft, pale yellowish tumour was found arising from the hypothalamus, surrounding the optic tracts and mammillary bodies and extending upwards between the layers of the septum pellucidum. The foramina of Monro were almost completely obstructed. Microscopically, the hypothalamic tumour proved to be a chronic granuloma consisting of lymphocytes, large and atypical histiocytes, giant cells and a small amount of pale, necrotic tissue. A single asteroid body was seen in one of the multinucleated giant cells. The pathological diagnosis was granuloma of undetermined aetiology, possibly sarcoid.

Although this case was eventually shown to have a lesion involving the brain extensively, the presenting mental picture over a period of at least three years was predominantly that of a functional mental illness. Only in the terminal phases of the disease were signs discovered that aroused suspicion of the underlying process. In retrospect, one wonders if the attending physician's observation of disorientation and confusion, and the wife's account that "he could not remember things from one hour to the next" might have raised the possibility of an organic psychosis rather than functional mental illness. However, an examining physician does not always find it a simple matter to assess orientation or memory functioning; for example, a patient's statement that his physician is a police agent may be an indication of delusional thinking rather than disorientation as to person in the usual meaning of the concept;

the claim that he forgets things may not be an indication of a fundamental defect of memory functioning but rather evidence of inattention, absorption in personal conflicts or distractability.

Excessive sleepiness is not uncommon in psychological illnesses and frequently is interpreted (and often probably correctly so) as an escape mechanism, but excessive sleepiness also can be an accompaniment of physical illnesses such as toxic states, lesions producing increased intracranial pressure, and in this particular patient may have been related to the site of the lesion which involved the hypothalamic area. It is interesting that this patient never had papilloedema even in the terminal stages, despite the presence of an extensive, infiltrating lesion of the brain producing internal hydrocephalus. The finding of normal optic discs certainly does not exclude a diagnosis of brain tumour. In this particular case, signs of organic mental symptoms were relatively few and difficult to evaluate. In fact the nature of the disease was only suspected when the general physical state made the diagnosis of schizophrenia no longer above question. This man was ill for more than three years. One wonders whether a more careful physical investigation sooner in the illness might have revealed physical abnormalities in their earliest stages.

These last three cases again illustrate the observation that an organic psychosis may present, for a time at least, as a functional mental illness. This observation is an important one as the examining physician may be led astray by not suspecting the presence of an organic lesion of the brain. Frequently, the functional mental picture is more apparent than real. In such cases more careful assessment of the mental state and more detailed physical investigation could cut down the incidence of "pure" functional mental pictures and shorten the period before organic mental symptoms are observed. These three cases, all with some features of dementia, are good examples of the variety of functional mental pictures which may obscure the underlying dementia. The first patient was depressed, the second ultimately assaulted his wife and was dealt with through the courts, while the third was considered to be schizophrenic. This theme forms the basis of the next chapter, "Functional mental illness associated with physical disease involving the brain."

Case 14

This spry, seventy-one year old farmer had been working and able to drive his car until four days before admission to the hospital in his home town. At that time he began to complain of dizziness and two days later it was noted that he was mentally confused and had difficulty finding his way about the home. The day before admission it was obvious that his memory was defective, his speech was slurred, the conversation difficult to follow and he could not carry out simple tasks such as tying his tie. Because of this deterioration in mental state he was admitted to hospital. In addition to this general deteriorated mental state there were times when he was very disorientated and disturbed, requiring restraint.

It was the opinion of the medical staff that they were probably dealing with a condition of cerebral arteriosclerosis and that certification to a mental hospital seemed a likely necessity. The family were very upset to learn of this opinion, were dissatisfied with the decision, signed his release from hospital against medical advice and took him at once to a general hospital in a larger centre.

Following the patient's admission to the second hospital, an interne interviewed the wife who supplied important additional information: (*a*) about three months ago, the patient began to complain of severe, steady, diffuse headaches; (*b*) two weeks ago he began to have difficulty in walking; (*c*) the patient had enjoyed good mental health until ten days ago when there was a sudden change as described above.

This sequence of events would be rather unusual for cerebral atherosclerosis resulting in widespread softenings, especially in the frontal regions. In this condition, the complaint of severe headache is not commonly made, and the onset of mental deterioration is not, as a rule, so sudden in a person who up until that time had good health. Furthermore, one would have expected a history of some localizing signs such as a mild hemiplegia or aphasia. As a matter of fact the physical findings were negative.

The interne, while not completely satisfied with a diagnosis of cerebral atherosclerosis, did not have sufficient findings to establish an alternative, but was concerned with the possibility of chronic subdural haematoma or frontal lobe tumour. During the next twenty-four hours the patient's mental state remained about the same: he thought he was still at home, gave his age as forty-two, was seven years wrong in the date of the year, at times was drowsy, and at other times exhibited perseveration. By the end of the second day in hospital his condition had deteriorated: he appeared more confused, was disorientated and had become incontinent and difficult to arouse. Plantar responses were now definitely extensor, pulse rate was slowed and there was some weakness of the grip of the left hand. Mild choking of the discs could be seen. At this time the house staff had become very concerned that the patient was suffering from an expanding intracranial lesion. There was no evidence of head injury nor was there a cranial bruit. An electroencephalogram was done and interpreted as a diffuse disorganization but without localizing signs. Skull X-rays revealed the fact that the pineal gland which was calcified was displaced approximately one centimetre downwards and posteriorly from its normal position but remained in the midline. This was interpreted as being strongly suggestive of a high frontoparietal lesion such as a subdural or extradural haematoma.

During the fourth night in hospital, the patient's responses became very limited, he was extremely drowsy and would only occasionally respond to stimulation. His pulse rate had decreased to 44 per minute with many premature beats and periods of pulsus alternans. The blood pressure had risen from 140/90 to 150/105 mm. Hg. A neurosurgical consultation was requested. At 1 A.M. the patient's condition was even worse. He had Cheyne-Stokes respiration. It was the consultant's opinion that they were dealing with a frontal lobe lesion on the right side, either a tumour or a subdural haematoma and that burr-holes should be made to clarify the diagnosis. This operation was immediately carried out. When the right burr-hole was made, a large clot was discovered which had liquefied and covered a portion of the frontal lobe. The thick membrane surrounding the clot was freed and opened in order to allow the brain which had been pushed ¾ of an inch away from the vault of the cranium to expand. The patient returned to the ward in an improved condition.

Postoperatively the patient did very well. His level of consciousness immediately improved and he was out of bed three days after the operation. For the first few postoperative days there was a mild degree of confusion and disorientation but this cleared completely by the time the patient was discharged on the ninth postoperative day. He was examined as an outpatient three weeks later, at which time he felt well enough to return to work, his mental state was completely normal and there were no abnormal physical findings.

This case illustrates a number of important principles. In the older age group, the presence of mental symptoms, whatever their nature may be, is often attributed to senile or atherosclerotic changes. While this may be correct in many cases, there is always the possibility of some underlying organic condition that could be corrected, as in the case under discussion.

Certain of the symptoms of this patient such as the periods of acute disturbance and disorientation are usually considered to be more typical of a delirium than a dementia. However, it is not uncommon for patients with dementia to have acute episodes of a delirious nature. This further illustrates the principle that we are dealing with syndromes or symptom patterns, and it is the predominating pattern that determines whether one makes a diagnosis of delirium or dementia. Many cases present no difficulty in that they are obviously delirious states or on the other hand states of dementia. But it is evident, as in psychiatric disorders generally, that there may be cases with overlapping features. Furthermore, there are instances in which a delirium may progress to a dementia. Also there are cases presenting as syndromes of dementia (e.g. case 19) which instead of following the usual course of permanent loss or increasing loss of mental functioning may get better.

3. INFECTION

Case 15

This patient, who worked as a butcher, enjoyed good health until the age of forty. At that time he began to vomit after breakfast and this continued almost daily for some months. The vomiting stopped, but during the following year, there was a gradual decline in sexual drive. One year before admission, that is two years after the period of vomiting, his wife noted that he was having some difficulty with speech, there was a tremor of his hands and his mental faculties began to fail. There was a gradual deterioration of memory, comprehension and orientation. He had frequent crying spells and was finally dismissed from his job.

These symptoms were thought to be due largely to long-standing friction between his wife and his brother's wife, who lived together under one roof. The constant discord was very upsetting to the patient and, although he tended to keep his feelings to himself, at times he expressed his concern.

It was the opinion of the attending psychiatrist that the condition was essentially a state of depression. The patient therefore was started on a course of electroconvulsive therapy at the out-patient department of a general hospital. After five treatments his memory became markedly worse; perseveration of behaviour and speech was in evidence. Electroconvulsive therapy was continued to a total of twenty treatments. His behaviour became more abnormal in that there were episodes of indecent exposure, but later a noticeable improvement set in three to four weeks after the termination of electroconvulsive therapy. He began to eat and sleep well, assisted his wife with some of the household tasks but was not well enough to return to work. About five months before admission he again began to vomit, always after meals. He was then referred to the out-patient department of a psychiatric hospital for another opinion. The examining psychiatrist noted a profound memory loss, difficulty with abstract thinking, emotional lability, perseveration and disconnected speech. This combination of mental symptoms, plus a definite tremor of the hands and a dysarthria, were the basis for the examining psychiatrist's diagnosis of a rather advanced organic psychosis. Accordingly, the patient was admitted to the in-patient department for further investigation.

In hospital, both assessment of the patient's personality from a developmental standpoint and further investigation of his physical state were instituted. The history disclosed that the patient had always been considered to be a stable person, but apart from this, no significant facts were gleaned. The physical examination did not contribute a great deal more than has already been mentioned, except for the presence of increased deep reflexes. The mental state was in keeping with fairly advanced dementia in that the patient was obviously confused, not knowing where he was, and his memory was very poor for both remote and recent events. There was a marked deterioration of personality, with untidiness, incontinence, inappropriate laughter and lack of emotional depth. The routine laboratory tests, including blood V.D.R.L. test,* were negative. The electroencephalogram showed generalized 3 to 6 per second slow waves, in keeping with fairly severe organic brain damage.

It seemed obvious that this was a case of organic psychosis in a stage of dementia. The question of causation was not clear. In fact, there were no leads in the history or in the mental or physical findings to indicate what factor or factors were responsible. Because of his age and the absence of localizing neurological signs and the negative laboratory findings, presenile dementia seemed the most likely diagnosis. Accordingly, an air encephalogram was done. To no one's surprise, the encephalogram indicated gross cerebral atrophy, with enlargement of the lateral and third ventricles and of the sulci. However, we were amazed to find that the cerebrospinal fluid obtained during the air study gave a very strongly positive Wasserman reaction, a colloidal gold reaction of 5555543210 and contained 116 mg. of protein per 100 ml. Our first reaction was that there had perhaps been a mistake in the identity of the spinal fluid and that this was the report on another patient. The reasons for not suspecting a paretic condition were the lack of a history of luetic infection or treatment, the absence of traces of bismuth in X-rays of the gluteal regions, the negative blood test for syphilis and the absence of rather characteristic neurological findings, such as Argyll Robertson pupils. The repeat examination of the cerebrospinal fluid confirmed the original report. The second testing of the blood gave a questionably positive V.D.R.L.

---

*The Venereal Disease Research Laboratory standard slide flocculation test is used in Ontario as a routine screening test of the blood for syphilis.

test, but the Wasserman test was done this time and found to be positive, as was also a treponema pallidum immobilization test.

Once satisfied that this was a case of paresis, we were curious to learn whether there was any corroborative history. The patient's wife was questioned carefully and she recalled that seven years previously, when they were about to be married in Saskatchewan, it was necessary for them to have a routine blood test. She stated that there was some delay in obtaining permission for marriage because there seemed to be something wrong with her husband's blood. She gave the name of the family doctor, whose records showed that there had been three doubtful Wasserman tests and the fourth blood test was negative.

The patient was treated with 900,000 units of penicillin in oil and aluminum monostearate three times weekly for six weeks but failed to respond to the treatment and continued to deteriorate mentally and physically. He died several months after the diagnosis was first established.

This case is helpful in illustrating a number of very important points that one may encounter in organic psychoses: The patient presented originally certain features compatible with functional mental illness, namely, a depressed state, for which he received electroconvulsive therapy and, as not infrequently happens, the depressed state was reversible and the patient improved. The improvement of the functional component of the mental illness often unmasks, or renders obvious, the organic mental symptoms, as it did in this particular case. Sometimes electroconvulsive therapy appears to even hasten the progress of the dementia.

This case also indicates the advisability of examination of cerebrospinal fluid in cases of organic psychosis in which the aetiological factors are obscure. Lumbar puncture not only established the diagnosis of paresis but also illustrated, once again, the fortunately rather rare occurrence in paresis of a negative serological test for syphilis but positive spinal fluid.

4. DEFICIENCY STATE

Case 16

A fifty-seven year old housewife was admitted to a general hospital and was stated by the relatives to have had good health until six weeks before, when she tripped and struck her head on the floor. Following this she complained of headache and weakness, felt unable to do any housework and remained in bed all the time. Two weeks before admission, her condition altered radically: she became confused, misidentified members of her family, and thought that her son long since dead was still alive; she vomited frequently and it was noted that her left eye turned inwards.

The family considered that she had been worrying a great deal recently about the birth of an illegitimate child to her daughter and by the necessity of moving from her home to a basement apartment.

On admission it was observed that, though she was co-operative, she was obviously confused and disoriented. She mistook some of the doctors for her dead son and talked about her son and daughter as though they were still living. Both recent and remote memory were poor. There was bilateral sixth nerve palsy, sluggish knee jerks and a left Babinski response was present. She was ataxic and there was deep muscle tenderness of the calves. The liver could be felt one finger's breadth below the right costal margin. The diagnosis favoured on admission was subdural haematoma, a diagnosis compatible with the history of head injury, headaches, rather sudden mental deterioration, sixth nerve palsies and a Babinski response. Another possibility, considered to be less likely, was cerebral thrombosis.

The following day it was felt that the patient had early papilloedema. On looking to the left, nystagmus could be elicited. Skull X-rays were normal. It was decided to investigate further the possibility of a subdural haematoma and accordingly burr holes were made in both sides of the skull but no subdural haematomata were found.

A consultant neurologist confirmed the presence of neurological abnormalities and altered mental state. It was known by this time that the protein of the cerebrospinal fluid was 60 mg. per 100 ml. and that the electroencephalogram was interpreted as indicating a mild, diffuse dysrhythmia. Although the pupils were not abnormal, the neurologist considered the possibility of an alcoholic encephalopathy of a mixed Wernicke's and Korsakoff's type. He felt that a brain stem tumour was very unlikely, since there was no seventh nerve involvement such as would be expected if a tumour were involving the nuclei of the sixth nerve. Large doses of a vitamin B complex were given daily.

In view of the consultant's opinion, a very careful questioning of the patient's family was undertaken. The relatives reluctantly admitted that the patient had been an alcoholic for the last ten years, consuming large quantities of beer, wine, whiskey and rum. Three years previously, her favourite daughter died and the patient drank even more heavily. Her fall, six weeks before admission, had followed a drinking bout. During the weeks immediately prior to admission, the family had been giving her up to twenty-six ounces of spirits daily "to keep her warm." This history of excessive intake of alcohol over a good many years made the diagnosis of alcoholic encephalopathy highly probable. In retrospect, certain of the signs might have raised the question of a state of thiamine deficiency, for example, the tender calves, the sluggish knee jerks and the fact that the liver was palpable.

The subsequent course of this patient's mental state is of interest, for it illustrates not only the degree of mental dysfunction which may occur in this condition, but also the amount of improvement that may occasionally take place.

During the next six weeks in hospital, the patient talked to herself much of the time. She stated that she had been to a staff doctor's office near by to have her picture taken. She said that she had spent two days with her grandchildren at her grandmother's house, when, in actual fact, she had not left the hospital. She said her own grandmother was in her 70's and saw nothing remarkable that she herself was 57. She was emotionally labile, laughing and crying on slight provocation. At times, she would be disturbed, unco-operative and wander about the ward bothering other patients.

At the time of discharge she was considered to be suffering from very severe dementia. On returning to the clinic a month later, she was still confused, denied that she had ever been in the habit of drinking alcoholic beverages and claimed she was still singing on the stage, as she had in her youth. Surprisingly, when she came to the clinic the following month, she was very much improved and answered questions about her surroundings and recent events quite rationally. She was seen repeatedly over the next two years, during which time she refrained from alcohol. The family stated that her memory had returned to normal and they considered her reasonably efficient about the house and "herself again." Detailed clinical assessment and psychological investigations were not done at this time, but it is highly likely that such procedures would have revealed a residual intellectual deficit.

5. CARDIOVASCULAR DISORDER

Case 17

This forty-nine year old man was transferred to a psychiatric hospital from a mental hospital where he had been for some six months. During the time in mental hospital, little information had been obtained from relatives, and the patient was uncommunicative. It seemed that, until about six years before, he had been a reliable factory worker, at which time he collapsed at work and was returned home in a confused state.

Since then he had been unable to work, and increasingly difficult to care for at home, which eventually necessitated his admission to the mental hospital. His behaviour in hospital raised the possibility of malingering, but the signs and symptoms were of such a nature that full investigation in a psychiatric hospital was considered advisable.

The examination by the admitting physician at the psychiatric hospital revealed a forty-nine year old man who looked considerably older and seemed markedly demented. He was disoriented as to time and place but knew who he was. He was apathetic and in answer to questions he would say, "I don't remember." His speech was slurred, saliva drooled from his mouth and he appeared to be blind.

Within a few days there was little doubt that this was essentially an organic psychosis rather than a functional illness or malingering. With regard to the type of organic psychosis, the following information indicated the presence of diffuse vascular disease:

(i) On admission, his blood pressure was 200/130 and on a previous admission to another hospital six years before was 150/100.

(ii) Thirteen years previously he had an episode of chest pain and breathlessness considered probably due to myocardial infarction because the electrocardiogram in the psychiatric hospital indicated old posterior myocardial infarction.

(iii) In the past he had had several episodes of numbness of the right side of the body, dizziness, vomiting, double vision and falling, for which he was admitted to general hospitals on three different occasions. On each occasion, there were neurological signs in keeping with a transient disorder of the brain stem.

(iv) The attacks of dizziness had increased in frequency, gait disturbance became apparent, and over a period of a year there was the gradual development of blindness.

Historical information obtained from relatives confirmed the presence of a dementing process which had been going on for at least four years. This took the form of increasing apathy, untidiness, impairment of recent memory, perseveration of speech and irrelevant conversation, to the point that he required complete care.

On detailed neurological examination, there was bilateral blindness with normal pupillary reactions to light and normal fundi, mild left facial weakness, slurring of speech, an apraxic gait, absent abdominal and cremasteric reflexes and a positive Oppenheim reflex on the left. These findings were compatible with, and suggestive of, widespread cerebral dysfunction, probably vascular in origin.

All laboratory tests were negative, with the exception of an elevated spinal fluid protein (86 mg. per 100 ml.) which is in keeping with brain degeneration.

In hospital, he gradually became more resistive, obstinate, hostile and threatening, for which he was given chlorpromazine. The next day he developed a right hemiplegia with aphasia (it is possible that there may have been a temporary fall in blood pressure following the administration of chlorpromazine). Within twenty-four hours he became semicomatose and quadriplegic. He lingered in this state, with some variability of his level of consciousness, for several months before death.

The findings in the brain at autopsy explained the clinical picture very well. There was widespread cerebral atherosclerosis, with multiple areas of softening and resultant loss of brain substance, the brain weighing only 990 grams. At their bifurcations both common carotid arteries were completely occluded by old, organized thrombi. There was a large area of softening in the cortical distribution of the right posterior inferior cerebellar artery, probably related to the episodes of dizziness, vomiting, double vision and falling mentioned in the history. There was very severe softening involving the complete distributions of the right anterior and middle cerebral arteries and extending backwards from the right frontal pole to the anterior part of the right occipital lobe. In the left cerebral hemisphere there was a large area of infarction in the distribution of the left middle cerebral artery. On the mesial surface of the left cerebral hemisphere could be seen a severe degree of softening in the cortical distribution of the left posterior cerebral artery. The location and extent of the areas of infarction explain the profound dementia, aphasia, blindness and paralyses. None of the lesions were of recent origin but they appeared to have been present for a considerable time.

Other findings at autopsy of interest were: an old, organized thrombus of the circumflex branch of the left coronary artery, which accounted for a healed infarct of the posterior wall of the left ventricle; generalized cardiac dilatation; nephrosclerosis. These post-mortem findings are in keeping with the history of chest pain, electrocardiographic abnormalities and recordings of hypertension over some years. (Again this case illustrates that the retinal vessels may be free of arteriosclerotic change although the cerebral vessels are severely affected.)

(Dr. J. B. McKay, Provincial Pathologist, Department of Health, Central Laboratory, Toronto, kindly supplied the description of the findings at post-mortem examination.)

6. ANOXIA

Case 18

This thirty year old housewife was admitted to hospital for a hysterectomy. Her general health had been good and she was described as having been well-adjusted. In preparation for the operation she was given a spinal injection of pontocaine, followed by a small amount of cyclopropane gas when the patient requested that she be put to sleep. Soon after the induction of anaesthesia she became apnoeic, ashen-grey and cyanosed. It was thought that her heart had stopped beating. Resuscitative measures included intubation, an intravenous injection of aminophylline, adrenaline injected into the heart and continuous administration of oxygen. The exact duration of the period of apnoea is uncertain. Finally, she began to breathe again and her general condition improved, but it was decided not to proceed with the operation. During the next two hours she received inhalations of carbon dioxide, and at the end of that time, the following signs were noted: rigidity of the extremities and rapid movements of the jaws; pupils unreactive to light; blood pressure 84/70 mm. Hg; pulse rate 112 per minute; respirations were irregular; the patient's colour was good and she was perspiring freely. During the next four hours there were occasional periods of spasticity of the neck, back and upper extremities with clenched fists and flaccid legs; the blood pressure fell to 80/30. By the end of this time, the blood pressure had risen to 100/74, the eyes were open with slight conjugate deviation to the right, the pupils were dilated and reacted sluggishly to light. The ocular fundi were normal. The respirations were slow and regular. The upper extremities were semi-flexed, rigid and resistant to movement. The abdominal and knee reflexes were absent but the ankle jerks were brisk. Babinski's and Brudzinski's signs were absent. There was some neck rigidity.

During the next few days, the patient gradually recovered from the stupor, the blood pressure and pulse rate returned to normal levels and the hypertonicity became intermittent. This improvement took place in the following stages: within twenty-four hours of the administration of the anaesthetic, corneal reflexes had returned, the patient began to groan and swallow occasionally, and at times yawn repeatedly with associated stretching movements; the knee jerks had become hyperactive. Two days following anaethesia, the patient responded to voices, was able to sip water, recognized her husband and called him by name. The conjugate deviation of the eyes had disappeared. On the third day she was able to converse in a weak voice.

Within two weeks it was obvious that the patient had sustained severe damage to the nervous system, with prominent symptoms of dementia. She was restless, confused, her memory was markedly impaired, her conversation was childish, at times she confabulated and exhibited a lack of judgment. Because of her mental state, she was transferred to a psychiatric hospital for further investigation and treatment.

At the time of admission to the psychiatric hospital, the physical examination was normal, except for slight ataxia of the hands and legs. During the first few weeks in hospital, the patient displayed the following manifestations of cerebral damage: in general, she seemed bewildered and was unable to recall events that had happened in recent months, particularly the circumstances of her admission to the general hospital, although she was quite capable of recalling events in her early life. She would wander about looking for her family in a slow, deliberate, mournful manner. She would talk at length in a rambling, disconnected manner of having been overseas recently; wondering if the war was over yet; would keep asking about her baby, as she seemed to be under the impression that she had just given birth to a baby; asked why she never had any visitors, although she was visited frequently by members of her family. She displayed considerable disorientation, being unable to name the hospital but thought it was in Toronto. She was unsure of the month or year, and even when informed of the date, she could only recall it for a few minutes. For the first few days, insight was negligible; however, later she began to display concern about her difficulty in remembering. She said that she was all right physically and kept asking, "What is wrong with me? Why can't I remember what's happened? How long will I be like this?"

Psychological investigations indicated marked confusion. During testing she spoke frequently of her "new-born infant" and this delusion persisted throughout each interview. On the Wechsler-Bellevue test her intelligence quotient was 79, a level thought to be much below her normal (her school record had been in keeping with a normal intelligence quotient). Other evidences of brain damage included a low score on the "digits reversed," on the block design, picture completion and digit symbol tests. In the Shipley-Hartford test the conceptual score of 71 indicated considerable intellectual impairment. Her memory quotient on the Wechsler Memory scale was 64, a score indicating considerable loss of memory.

An electroencephalogram recorded three weeks after the episode of anoxia was abnormal with much slow wave activity and instability of pattern. The abnormalities were generalized and bilaterally synchronous. The second tracing, a week later, indicated slight improvement, the alpha rhythm of the occipital lobes being more stable in rate and amplitude. However, evidence of abnormal activity chiefly of a paroxysmal nature could be seen. Further tracings made during the stay in hospital were similar but with an added finding of occasional bursts of slow waves originating from the right frontotemporal region.

One year after discharge from hospital, the patient was seen again in the out-patient department to observe her progress. She had resumed the duties of a housewife but continued to show loss of memory, emotional lability, apathy and lack of initiative. She displayed some awareness of her inadequacies but, none the less, was optimistic because she noticed some improvement in mental functioning. The psychological tests were repeated with results which were similar but perhaps slightly better than the year before. The electroencephalographic patterns were those of episodic 5 to 6 per second slow wave activity, particularly in the frontal areas.

Recently, that is ten years after the illness, she was again examined. The patient continued to be aware of her poor memory and to worry sometimes about her loss of efficiency as a housewife. She had been carrying on a fairly normal existence at home, but was unable to shop without a list and avoided visiting relatives in the city for fear she would lose her way. Events she could not remember included her illness ten years previously; an admission to another hospital four months before; and an explanation made to her by the doctor twenty minutes before her interview. Her husband described her as being irritable and subject to tantrums. In general, she appeared apathetic and, at times, mildly depressed.

The same psychological tests were administered and the results indicated over-all improvement with, however, persistent impairment of both memory and the ability to conceptualize. The results of the tests are recorded in the following table:

Interval after anoxia	Wechsler-Bellvue intelligence	Shipley-Hartford	Wechsler memory
A few weeks	79	71	64
One year	85	71	62
Ten years	92	79	83

The electroencephalograph ten years after the episode of anoxia was interpreted as normal. A few months before the ten year follow-up examination, the patient had been studied in another hospital because she had severe headaches. At that time an air encephalogram was reported to be within normal limits. She was considered to be suffering from a reactive depression for which she was given three electroshock treatments with considerable subsequent improvement.

While this case presented no difficulty in diagnosis, it does illustrate how devastating can be the effect of a relatively brief period of anoxia on the functioning of cerebral cells. It also shows that considerable improvement may be expected in some cases, probably from a combination of better functioning of the damaged cerebral cells and as a result of a relearning process. In this patient the improvement has occurred in spite of increasing age which is usually accompanied by some decrease in mental efficiency.

7. METABOLIC DISORDER

Case 19

This fifty-seven year old woman had been treasurer of a religious organization for many years and was considered to be a very valuable employee, because of her exactness in carrying out these duties. However, those about her had gradually come to realize that she was making mistakes in the accounting, that her memory was failing, and in general, that she was mentally slow and, at times, confused. Furthermore, her family were becoming increasingly worried because she would wander away from home, and on return, would be unable to tell where she had been. Eventually, her efficiency at work deteriorated to the point that the employers were giving her less and less work to do. At times, she would not come in to work, and latterly was encouraged by her employers not to come. In spite of these symptoms, no attempt was made to consult a physician.

While visiting a relative in another city, the patient was persuaded to undergo a medical examination. Fortunately, the physician she consulted investigated the problem in a methodical manner, commencing by taking a thorough history. Of significance in this history was the fact that she had had a thyroidectomy twelve years previously, and within several weeks following this operation she had had a typical grand mal seizure. Similar seizures had occurred at intervals from that time on. The family had been so sensitive about these episodes that they had discouraged her from consulting a doctor. The history of a thyroidectomy, followed by epileptic seizures, raised the possibility of hypoparathyroidism in the mind of the examining physician. This diagnosis was further supported by the history that her vision had become so bad within three years following the thyroidectomy that she had to have cataracts removed bilaterally. On physical examination, the only abnormalities were a positive Chvostek's sign and transverse ridging of the finger nails. The mental state was one of bewilderment; the ability to remember recent and remote events was impaired. She lacked any insight into her state, feeling quite capable of resuming her work although she was obviously incapable of doing arithmetical calculations. As a result of the history and examination carried out in his office, the doctor made a provisional diagnosis of hypoparathyroidism. For further confirmation he had the serum calcium measured and the result was 7.5 mg. per 100 ml.; this finding was in keeping with the diagnosis. His advice was that the patient should return home and consult a doctor in her own city. He sent a report of his findings to this physician.

On return home, the patient was promptly admitted to hospital, where the mental and physical findings were confirmed. The serum calcium was 4.6 mg. and the serum phosphorus was 5.1 mg. per 100 ml. There was prolongation of the Q-T interval in the electrocardiogram. In repeated electroencephalographic tracings one could see bursts of bilaterally symmetrical, high-voltage, three per second waves. Skull films were normal, including lack of any evidence of intracranial calcification.

As treatment for the hypoparathyroidism she was given dihydrotachysterol (A.T.10) and a diet high in calcium, with a supplement of calcium chloride. With this treatment the whole general condition improved. She became mentally alert with improvement of memory and return of her ability to calculate. The Chvostek's sign disappeared, serum calcium rose to normal levels and the electrocardiogram also reverted to normal. (This is an example of the way in which electrocardiograms may reflect ionic abnormalities, particularly those of calcium or potassium.) There was improvement in the electroencephalogram, although minimal signs of abnormality persisted.

Six weeks following admission she was discharged to her home. Medication consisted of vitamin D, a high calcium diet, and in addition, she was to take dilantin for an indefinite period. She resumed her work as treasurer and has continued to function efficiently for the last six years.

While this case may appear to have been simple and straightforward from the point of view of diagnosis, it might have been a very confusing picture if the examining physician had not approached the diagnosis in a methodical manner. He first obtained a detailed history which immediately gave him leads, and because of sound clinical knowledge, he was able to make full use of these leads. On the basis of an office examination only, he was able to confirm this initial opinion by having the serum calcium determined.

This case also illustrates another important principle: in some instances, signs and symptoms of dementia may diminish markedly, suggesting that many of the cerebral cells have not been damaged irreparably but were only temporarily functioning inefficiently. If the underlying disorder can be corrected, for example, by treating a metabolic disturbance such as hypoparathyroidism, or by treating an infection before the cerebral cells have been permanently damaged, as in an early case of general paresis, recovery may be quite dramatic. Perhaps this fact is not widely enough known. Certainly, lay people, such as the relatives of the patient under discussion, often hesitate to seek medical help because they feel that nothing can be done. Sometimes doctors, too, will diagnose dementia without making a strong effort to determine the cause because they think that all patients with dementia have a poor prognosis. The reader will note that case 14 (p. 116) is another example of a patient exhibiting some features of dementia in whom removal of the cause resulted in marked improvement.

(We are indebted to Dr. R. C. Dickson, Professor of Medicine, Dalhousie University, formerly Physician-in-Chief of the Wellesley Division, Toronto General Hospital, for permission to publish this case.)

8. TRAUMA AND OTHER SETTINGS FOR DEMENTIA

Not uncommonly severe injury to the head, for example occurring as a result of an automobile accident, is followed by dementia. In such cases there is little doubt about the relationship between the injury and the mental deterioration. Occasionally a boxer who has fought many times and perhaps been "knocked out" frequently will present with mild to moderate dementia.

It is a common observation that some patients who have suffered repeated epileptic attacks, especially if the seizures began in childhood, show evidence of dementia. Some clinicians feel that very extensive and repeated courses of electroconvulsive therapy apparently damage the brain of certain individuals and give rise to blunting of higher cerebral functioning.

Interestingly enough, although many toxic substances including a variety of drugs give rise to delirious states, very few produce dementia. Alcohol is one of the common exceptions if taken in large quantities over many years. Whether the deleterious effect of chronic alcoholism on the functioning of cerebral cells is due entirely to nutritional deficiencies or in part to a direct effect of alcohol, is still a debatable point. Of other toxic substances which sometimes produce dementia, lead may be mentioned.

CHAPTER XIV

Functional Mental Illness Associated with Physical Disease Involving the Brain

Occasionally, functional psychiatric syndromes are associated with organic disorders involving altered functioning of brain tissue, for example, a schizophrenic illness in an individual with a luetic infection of the central nervous system (G.P.I.—general paresis). It is customary in these cases, if there is apparently a causal relationship between the physical disorder and the psychiatric disorder, to consider the organic disease of the brain as merely one factor in releasing a psychiatric syndrome determined by the patient's basic personality pattern. Because of the danger that a functional psychiatric syndrome may imply to the unwary clinician that there is no organic involvement of the brain, the authors have included examples of such associated conditions in this book on organic psychoses to assist the clinician in his efforts to make a correct diagnosis. Furthermore, if the physical condition is corrected, frequently the psychiatric condition improves or completely disappears. If the physical disorder progresses, the symptoms typical of an organic mental illness usually make their appearance eventually.

Case 20: *Involutional Psychosis and Myxoedema*

Two weeks before admission to a psychiatric hospital, this patient, aged forty-three, developed definite mental symptoms. She awoke at 1 A.M. claiming that her house was being broken into and later telling her friends that police were going to search the house. She was also concerned that someone was trying to steal money from her purse. This anxious, fearful state worsened until she appeared to be dazed and very tired. On one occasion she awoke at 3 A.M. and insisted there were two men and a woman on the porch. She was taken to a general hospital for observation where she was considered to be suffering from involutional melancholia. Because she was so resistive, refusing food and struggling with the nurses, it was considered necessary to admit her to a psychiatric hospital.

On admission to the psychiatric hospital, she appeared bewildered, was very quiet, somewhat resistive and at times was very lethargic, appearing mentally retarded. She described auditory hallucinations, would become apprehensive, and stated that she wished to see a detective about some private business. She was rather pale with a high flush on her cheek, the skin was dry and there were irregular, exfoliating plaques on both forearms. There was some non-pitting oedema of the eyelids, hands and feet. The hair was coarse and the lips had a smooth coral colour. The voice was hoarse. No thyroid enlargement was present. The temperature was 98° F. The haemoglobin was 9.8 g. per 100 ml. (63 per cent), the red blood count 2.9 million per c. mm. and most of the red cells were large and well-filled, with however more variation in size and shape than is normally found. The white blood count, non-protein nitrogen, van den Bergh reaction and Wasserman tests were all normal.

These physical findings, namely the pallor, malar flush, smooth coral lips, coarse dry hair, hoarse voice and the slowness of mental activity were typical of myxoedema. The basal metabolic rate was minus 42 per cent.

Further investigation of the history indicated that the patient had been a well-adjusted woman until recently. For the last three years she had had a great deal of worry over an irresponsible daughter who became pregnant before marriage and soon after marriage had two more children in rapid succession. Two months before the patient was admitted to hospital she was obliged to take into her home her daughter and children. About this time the daughter's eldest child became ill with otitis media complicated by facial paralysis and had to go to hospital. Shortly after this the patient's daughter was admitted to hospital for confinement. The patient had a great deal to do managing the house, visiting the hospital, and later looking after both convalescent patients when they were able to leave hospital. In addition to these responsibilities, the patient found the noisiness and lack of discipline of the children very trying. Furthermore, she refused to give up her outside activities in spite of the fact that she was feeling more and more fatigued. This symptom was part of a progressive state of ill-health over the previous two years in which there had been a gain in weight, menorrhagia, anaemia, oedema and a gradual slowing of activity. It was not until two weeks before admission that serious mental symptoms appeared as mentioned above.

Desiccated thyroid grains one-half was given daily. In about two weeks the skin was less dry, the myxoedematous patches on the arms were disappearing, the patient was brighter and free from any psychiatric symptoms. She was discharged one month after admission much improved in every way.

Although the psychological and social factors were undoubtedly of major importance in this mental breakdown, the physical disturbance certainly must have contributed. Fatigue and lack of drive are rather characteristic of myxoedema and these symptoms lower one's ability to deal with problems of living, which in this case were excessive. Furthermore, there is considerable evidence from the work of various investigators to indicate that in myxoedema the cells of the brain are not functioning optimally. This last factor must contribute significantly to the difficulties of the individual in coping with stress.

Case 21: Psychoneurosis and Porphyria

This twenty year old girl was the youngest of four daughters in a family of Ukrainian parentage. There were no significant family illnesses. The girl's mother was an overprotective, domineering woman and as a child the patient was quiet, reserved and lacking in self-confidence. She completed Grade X at age 17 and worked in factories. She was married at age 18 to a skilled labourer four years her senior. This marriage took place against strong objection by her mother. There were also emotional problems involving a change in religion and fear of the responsibilities of parenthood. She soon became pregnant and her first child died shortly after birth. Some months later she attempted to abort herself.

The illness which finally led to admission to hospital began with fatigue, severe abdominal pain and numbness and tingling of the extremities. She was admitted to a general hospital but was unmanageable, throwing herself about, wanting to go home to her mother and behaving in a most unco-operative way. At that time a number of physicians thought the problem was psychogenic. After two months in the general hospital she was certified as mentally ill and admitted to a mental hospital.

On admission, she was restless, drowsy, dehydrated, with sunken eyes. The admission blood pressure was 155/92 mm. Hg. The physician who first examined her obtained a history that her urine had been "very dark red" for a year. Soon after admission the urine was observed to be a "dark port-wine" colour. Neither the laboratory of the mental hospital nor of a general hospital was able to identify the source of this colour. It is not known whether a specimen of dark-coloured urine was tested. Because of the inability to demonstrate porphyrins at this time, the possibility of porphyria was not seriously considered again until just before death. The patient was found to be about 8 weeks pregnant. Physical examination and investigations of the blood, urine and spinal fluid were negative. Chest X-ray was negative and the level of non-protein nitrogen was 38 mg. per 100 ml. The psychiatric differential diagnosis was psychoneurosis—mixed type or schizophrenia, with the former diagnosis being favoured.

For the first little while in hospital the patient thought the voices of other patients were those of her mother and sisters. Later she realized that she had been mistaken and that it was part of her sickness.

Within a week or two after admission, the patient was much more co-operative and except for complaints about various pains in the abdomen and extremities, which were interpreted as being of psychogenic origin, her mental state was not abnormal. This general mental picture remained pretty well unchanged until her death five months after admission.

After several weeks in hospital she developed hoarseness. A further physical examination one month after admission disclosed that while she had been losing weight generally, from 140 lbs. down to 110 in recent months, the weight loss seemed to have affected certain regions in particular. There was definite wasting and atrophy in the scapulohumeral group of muscles and also some weakness and wasting in the muscles of the pelvic girdle. The sternomastoid and trapezius muscles were not involved and the muscles of the forearm were comparatively intact. She was unable to raise her hands as high as her head, but the grip of the hands was fairly strong. There was no noticeable weakness of the facial muscles of expression. The tongue showed no weakness or wasting and the ocular movements were normal. There was no loss of sensation anywhere to light touch, pin-prick, heat, cold or position. The reflexes were slightly decreased. There was paralysis of the left vocal cord. It was felt that the physical condition was either motor neurone disease or muscular dystrophy. These more recent physical findings involving the peripheral nerves and muscles were not thought to be related to the mental illness. There was no further progression in her illness until the fourth month in mental hospital, when she developed persistent vomiting lasting more than a week and requiring intravenous medication. The pregnancy appeared to be progressing normally.

There was no further advancement of her illness until several days before death, when she became noticeably weaker and developed bronchopneumonia. At this time the presence of marked muscle wasting and weakness compatible with a severe peripheral neuritis raised again the possibility of porphyria, and when the urine was tested on the day of death it was found to contain porphyrins.

Post-mortem examination of the central nervous system was essentially negative. There were slight changes in some of the nerve roots, consisting of early breakdown of myelin sheaths with the presence of some fat globules and histiocytes between the fibres.

In summary, the following facts were of significance: A number of personal problems around the time of the patient's marriage and first pregnancy appear to have been very stressful to her and her behaviour became such that she eventually was admitted first to a general hospital and then to a mental hospital. The admitting physician at the mental hospital, on obtaining a history of dark urine, abdominal pain, paraesthesias in the extremities and mental illness, had the urine tested but no porphyrins were reported to be present. The subsequent findings of peripheral neuropathy with patchy muscular wasting and the positive test for porphyrins on the day of death together with the history of dark urine and the complaints of abdominal pain, paraesthesias and transient mental symptoms all pointed to the likelihood of porphyria. It is probable that the excretion of porphyrins in the urine was intermittent, as it is in many cases of porphyria, and had the urine been tested repeatedly, the diagnosis might well have been established at an earlier stage of the illness.

Case 22: Schizophrenic Reaction and General Paresis

This patient, aged thirty-two, came to a psychiatric hospital on the advice of a physician as she felt that there was something the matter and wished to get her difficulties straightened out. She expressed concern that men were especially interested in her, that her employer was in love with her, had hypnotized her and had sent electric currents through her. This embarrassing situation had led to her dismissal from work.

It was learned from reliable informants that the patient had always been very quiet, reserved, sensitive and not a good mixer. Four months before admission there was a gradual change in her personality, finally culminating in the symptoms which led to her dismissal. She was very disturbed about this and said that it was for political reasons. She kept writing to the manager asking him to correct the whole situation. In addition, she started reading books on psychology and hygiene as she felt there might be "something the matter with me." Later she consulted a physician who advised admission to a psychiatric hospital.

On admission, physical examination including full neurological examination revealed no abnormality. In hospital she appeared preoccupied, was seclusive and untidy in her personal appearance. At times she would express her paranoidal ideas at length but often her conversation would be vague and difficult to understand.

The history, mental picture and the lack of physical findings were all in keeping with a rather typical paranoid schizophrenic illness. However, to the surprise of the attending staff, the routine blood sample was reported as giving a positive Kahn reaction. A lumbar puncture was then done and the cerebrospinal fluid Wasserman was found to be four-plus, the Kahn two-plus, protein 52 mg. per 100 ml. and the colloidal gold reaction 4432210000. As a result of these laboratory findings, further inquiries were made about a past history of venereal infection. The patient stated that some four years previously she had had a rash but that an examination of the blood at that time was negative.

In view of the undoubted evidence of paretic infection, it was considered that the schizophrenic illness was probably related to the luetic infection. Treatment for the paretic condition was instituted, and within a matter of weeks, the disordered mental state had subsided. She had become tidy in her appearance, was more sociable and displayed good insight into her condition.

Case 23: Manic State and General Paresis

A thirty-two year old woman was admitted to a psychiatric hospital being very talkative, excited, euphoric, unco-operative and irritable. She was extremely distractible, made personal remarks and presented the general picture of a manic illness. There was no evidence of hallucinations, delusions or disorientation. Investigation of this woman's history indicated that she had always been quiet and friendly and had shown no untoward behaviour. About six weeks before admission she had some teeth extracted, following which she complained of being extremely tired at work. Two weeks before admission she developed a cold. There was still some infection around the teeth and she had a fever. She became restless, talkative and excited. Her behaviour became so unusual that her employer thought she was intoxicated. Three days before admission she became quite argumentative, would go out on the street and talk to strangers. She finally became quite unmanageable, smashing lamps in the house and behaving in such a noisy and destructive manner that it was necessary to admit her to hospital.

All physical findings, including neurological, were normal except for occasional slight slurring of speech which was considered to be due to heavy sedation. As in the previous case, the mental state, including the absence of memory defect, disorientation or other signs of organic mental illness, together with the history of the development of the illness and the normal physical findings were in keeping with a functional mental illness, in this instance a manic state. Again, as in the previous case, a positive Wasserman and Kahn reaction was found in the routine examination of the blood. A spinal puncture was then done and the fluid contained thirty-six cells per c. mm. and a protein concentration of 89 mg. per 100 ml.; Wasserman and Kahn reactions were positive and the colloidal gold curve was 5554332100.

She was treated for the paretic condition and improved rapidly. Two months after beginning treatment she appeared to be fully recovered, being quiet and pleasant, sleeping well and displaying good insight.

Active syphilitic infections appear to be decreasing in frequency with the result that routine serological tests are no longer carried out in some hospitals. The last two cases illustrate how important the laboratory tests may be in the diagnosis of unsuspected active syphilis. Neither of the patients had symptoms of delirium or dementia, nor did they have physical signs of syphilitic disease. Only the blood tests provided a clue to the diagnosis.

In the authors' opinion, these last two cases are especially helpful in illustrating this third group of syndromes, namely functional mental illnesses associated with organic diseases of the brain. Both patients had evidence of paretic infection of the brain yet one presented a classical picture of schizophrenia, the other a typical example of manic illness. Some clinicians would prefer to consider both cases as general paresis even though the mental symptoms were functional in character and devoid of any of the symptoms usually considered pathognomonic of organic psychoses such as memory loss or disorientation.

It might be argued that while both patients had the same type of infection, the anatomical distribution of the damage to the brain brought about by the spirochaetes might vary considerably in the two cases: for example, one patient might have extensive damage in the region of the hypothalamus while the other patient had little involvement of this area. Could not such differences in involvement result in rather major differences in the clinical mental picture? Alternatively, if a more detailed psychological and psychiatric investigation had been carried out, it is quite possible that there would have been indications in the development and structure of the personalities which would have helped explain why one patient, under the additional stress of damage to the central nervous system, broke down with a schizophrenic reaction whereas the other, with a similar disease of the brain, broke down with a manic illness. If the clinician prefers to view such cases in this manner he is less apt to think of such patients as "cases of paresis" but as two individuals with different personalities developing two forms of functional mental illness, the infection being an important but not the only major factor in the causation complex.

Case 24: *Hysteria and Sydenham's Chorea*

This eighteen year old patient was attending the prenatal clinic of a general hospital. Two months before term she became very concerned about the pregnancy and it was considered that this concern was exaggerated and out of keeping with the circumstances. She phoned the hospital a number of times in an agitated state complaining of abdominal cramps. Because of this, she was admitted to hospital, it being considered that she might be having labour pains.

On admission, the patient was observed to move constantly, tossing about in bed with writhing movements of the hands and arms, kicking of the legs, twisting of the trunk and marked facial grimacing. It was the impression of the examining physician that the clinical picture was essentially a psychoneurotic reaction. This appeared to be confirmed by the fact that these movements ceased for a short time when the patient was asked to control them. Furthermore, a complete physical examination revealed no abnormality. The mother, on being interviewed, stated that for the past week she had noticed that the patient had been swinging her right leg outward when walking and that her right arm had become clumsy. The patient had been very concerned about any mild pain during the pregnancy and the day before admission was so disturbed, restless and crying that her husband could not talk with her. On two occasions the patient attacked her husband when he disagreed with her. For the most part, this description given by the mother seemed further evidence indicating a neurotic reaction with hysterical features.

However, in the next few days, she became more and more disturbed and despite heavy sedation she continued to be extremely hyperactive. The staff were so concerned about the possibility of injury that her mattress was placed on the floor and her bed removed. During this period the temperature rose to 106° F. These new developments forced a reconsideration of the diagnosis of hysteria and a renewed search for physical findings.

The spinal fluid and skull films were quite normal. There was evidence of mild, diffuse dysrhythmia in the electroencephalogram. It was impossible to assess her mental functioning in detail but she was obviously confused, expressed some bizarre ideas, and at times would not respond to questions. She was examined by a neurological consultant who was impressed by the type of involuntary movements of the patient and considered them so typical of chorea that he strongly favoured the possibility of the patient having Sydenham's chorea. At the height of the illness, she gave birth to a stillborn seven months' foetus. Over a period of three weeks, the choreiform movements and the acute mental disturbance subsided, but there remained marked emotional lability and general irritability. Her family signed her out of hospital. The staff were agreed on a diagnosis of Sydenham's chorea.

It is known that when Sydenham's chorea occurs during pregnancy, the disease may take a fulminating course, and in such circumstances the term chorea gravidarum is used. Early in the illness, emotional instability is commonly noted and this may be the first indication of underlying disease of the nervous system. In this particular case the initial mental symptoms were functional in nature and the motor disturbance was erroneously considered to be part of an hysterical illness. Later, features of delirium and chorea made their appearance.

Case 25: Behaviour Disorder and Huntington's Chorea
We found the following case most interesting as it illustrates a number of pitfalls that may be encountered by physicians in dealing with the particular group of patients described in this chapter. In some of these cases which present as functional psychiatric syndromes, psychological and social factors seem obviously responsible for the pattern. As a result of the obviousness of these factors, the physician is more likely to fail to suspect the possibility of an organic disease of the brain contributing to the clinical picture. This particular case, since it presented as a behaviour disorder, came to the attention of social agencies for some years before the patient reached a medical clinic.

The patient, a teen-age girl, had been a concern to her father for several years and had been taken by him to different agencies because of incorrigibility, inability to keep a job, association with undesirable companions and promiscuous behaviour, culminating in an illegitimate pregnancy. These agencies included the Big Sisters, the Y.W.C.A. and the Juvenile Court. This was the presenting situation when the girl's father brought her to a psychiatric clinic at the age of eighteen. Such behaviour is a frequent reason for referral to social agencies, family physicians and psychiatric clinics. On assessment of the early and recent environment, the behaviour of the patient often appears understandable in the light of the story of broken homes and lack of affection and discipline that are so frequent in cases of this type.

In this instance the obvious psychosocial factors were as follows: The girl's mother had also been an unstable person in her early years to the point that she had been admitted to a mental hospital when the patient was two years of age. From that age on the child not only lacked a mother, but heard from time to time that her mother was mentally ill and that there were other members of the family who were also mentally ill. The father was evidently a rather inadequate person and unable to maintain a stable home. As a result, the patient was brought up in a number of foster homes. She was very happy for some years with a foster mother with whom she lived until the age of fourteen. This foster mother became ill and the girl had to be placed elsewhere. It was from then on that her behaviour became progressively more of a problem.

The examining physician, on pursuing the question of the mother's mental illness, learned that the mother also had had an early history of emotional instability, promiscuity and stealing. She eventually attempted suicide on a number of occasions, was admitted to a psychiatric hospital twice, and on the basis of the mental illness and concomitant physical findings, her condition was diagnosed Huntington's chorea. She was certified to a mental hospital where she died fifteen years later at the age of thirty-seven. This information directed the attention of the physician to a detailed family history and raised the possibility in his mind that his patient might also be suffering from the same disease. It was learned that the maternal great-grandfather had symptoms which strongly suggested the diagnosis of Huntington's chorea and the maternal grandfather was definitely diagnosed **Huntington's** chorea. From the age of thirty to forty-five he was described as having had involuntary movements of hands, face and arms. He was irritable, had outbursts of temper and fits of depression, and committed suicide at the age of forty-five. The mother of the patient had five siblings: a brother committed suicide at age eighteen; a sister, who suffered from epilepsy, died at age nineteen in a mental hospital; another brother, age forty-five, has Huntington's chorea.

Further historical information of importance included the fact that for the previous six months involuntary movements of various parts of the body, described by her father as "twitchings," had been observed. There was also a noticeable change in her ability to speak.

On examination, dysarthria, involuntary movements of the limbs and eyelids, ataxia and inco-ordination were quite noticeable. Her judgment was limited but there were no definite signs of organic mental impairment on clinical examination. She was admitted to a psychiatric hospital for full investigation. Psychological studies revealed the following: "The patient reaches an intelligence quotient of 75 on the Wechsler-Bellevue Scale. As she is known to have had an intelligence quotient of 91 when tested seven years previously, this indicates a definite impairment of functioning. Diminished concentration, attention, pattern perception and ability to learn new material are considered indicative of intellectual impairment of an organic nature." The electroencephalogram was reported as follows: "This is a moderately abnormal E.E.G. with a high content of four to seven per second slow waves of average amplitude appearing rather diffusely over the cerebral cortex." The radiologist interpreted the air encephalogram as evidence of brain degeneration involving the frontal lobes.

It was the opinion of the hospital staff that she should be transferred to a mental hospital. The father did not wish to do so and took her home. Three months later, the father requested assistance in having his daughter admitted to a mental hospital. She had resumed her promiscuous behaviour, was not working, and had become incontinent of urine in public. Arrangements were then made for her admission to mental hospital.

Three years later, the mental hospital reported that there had been a gradual decrease in her ability to concentrate and think clearly. The physical symptoms had progressed markedly to the point where the patient had great difficulty in walking and frequently stumbled and fell.

This case is not only another example of the association of a functional psychiatric disorder and organic disease of the brain, but raises a number of questions. In the early stages of this behaviour disorder, were psychological and social forces largely, if not completely, responsible for the psychiatric pattern? Does a genetic disease of the central nervous system such as Huntington's chorea render the individual more susceptible to this type of behaviour disorder? If the genetic factor did not predispose to emotional instability in the early stages, at what stage did it begin to be of significance? Certainly it would be difficult to discount the organic dysfunctioning of the brain as an important factor by the time the patient was first seen in clinic.

Case 26: Schizophrenia Associated with ACTH Therapy for Nephrosis

Although the following case does not present a diagnostic problem, it illustrates a functional mental illness developing in the course of a physical disorder which was being treated with ACTH. As functional syndromes are not uncommonly the presenting picture in mental illnesses associated with ACTH and adrenal steroid therapy, they can mislead the attending physician if he is not aware that the patient is receiving this treatment or fails to recognize the possible relationship between the medication and the mental illness.

This twenty-one year old Chinese patient had been attending the out-patient department of a general hospital over a period of a year. When first examined, he had a four-plus albuminuria, casts in the urine, a blood pressure of 128/118 mm. Hg and a left pleural effusion. On conservative treatment he improved moderately for a few months but generalized oedema with ascites developed and he was therefore admitted to hospital.

Examination on admission revealed bilateral pleural effusions, oedema up to the waist and shifting dullness in the abdomen. The blood pressure was 110/80 mm. Hg. The urine contained four-plus albumin, hyaline, granular and cellular casts and red and white blood cells. The specific gravity ranged between 1.005 and 1.013. The level of non-protein nitrogen in the blood was normal, serum cholesterol 710 mg. per 100 ml. and serum albumin reduced to 2.1 g. per 100 ml. These findings were compatible with a diagnosis of the nephrotic phase of chronic glomerulonephritis.

After a few weeks' treatment in hospital he had failed to improve and it was decided to give daily infusions of ACTH intravenously. With this therapy he improved markedly; the albuminuria decreased and sometimes the urine was free of albumin; the serum cholesterol fell to 251 mg. per 100 ml. and the serum albumin rose to 4.9 g. per 100 ml.; he had a marked diuresis, voiding between three and four litres of urine a day; the pleural effusions, ascites and peripheral oedema disappeared. ACTH was accordingly given only every three days. Although the nephrotic state had improved dramatically, six weeks after the beginning of the ACTH therapy the patient became very apprehensive and suddenly attempted to cut his throat with a mirror. Since it has been observed repeatedly that ACTH therapy may precipitate a mental illness, this medication was promptly discontinued. In the next few days he expressed the thought that people were trying to kill him and that people on the radio were telling him to go home. At times he was unresponsive, failing to answer questions. Five days after cessation of the ACTH therapy the patient's mental state improved considerably but not completely. It was noted by the family and the physicians over the next few months that he was seclusive, laughed inappropriately at times, expressed some confused thoughts about devils and failed to resume his social and work activities.

Although detailed information about this patient's previous personality make-up was not available, there had been no overt signs of psychosis either during the year of attending the out-patient department or during the weeks in hospital prior to the treatment with ACTH. However, the fact that the patient's mental state did not return to normal poses the likelihood that in this patient there was a strong predisposition to schizophrenic illness.

Case 27: Schizophrenic Illness Associated with a Metabolic Disturbance of Unknown Nature (Periodic Catatonia)

The following case is introduced especially because it raises some points of major theoretical interest. These will be discussed after describing the case.

The patient, aged twenty-eight, has a family history indicating considerable emotional instability. The maternal grandfather was an alcoholic, the mother had suffered from involutional melancholia and two maternal uncles committed suicide. The father was also an alcoholic and one brother was mentally defective, epileptic, and died at the age of seven.

The patient had been an intelligent, competent, skilled worker, although somewhat shy and dependent. At the age of twenty-two, he suddenly developed the first signs of mental illness. He had been working as a lineman for a telephone company. He did not return home from work but went to the house of a friend. His behaviour seemed strange and the friend went to the patient's father asking him to come for his son. However, by the time they had reached the friend's home, the patient had left the house and was said to be walking in his stocking feet and carrying a rifle. He was found walking about in a dazed manner, and after getting into the car began to cry. He appeared very exhausted and bewildered. The family physician was called and it was his opinion that the patient should be in a mental hospital. A second physician was of the same opinion and the patient was admitted to a mental hospial. The doctors noted the following mental state: "confused, alternately quiet and restless; pounds his head and says his head is made of wood, that it is completely solid so that he cannot think; waxy flexibility elicited; recently has become seclusive, irritable and cries at times."

In the mental hospital the symptoms were considered typical of a catatonic type of schizophrenia. After several months in hospital, during which time he received electroconvulsive therapy, he was discharged as "recovered." He resumed work with the telephone company but it was soon evident that he was not well. He had several disturbed phases of short duration: for a few days he would remain away from work, lying in bed staring into space, mute and inactive. Two years after his first serious illness, while working in another city, he devolped rather quickly the same sequence of symptoms and was admitted to another mental hospital. Again he was diagnosed schizophrenia, catatonic type, and was stated to have improved dramatically after one electroshock treatment. Within a matter of days the catatonic state recurred, and he went through a series of these illnesses over the following few months. At first, he was treated with electroconvulsion, but in view of the recurring nature of the illness it was decided to observe the rhythm of the symptoms. It was noted that partial recovery would occur spontaneously after about eight or nine days of catatonic stupor and last for about the same length of time. It was concluded that this was probably a case of the periodic catatonia type of schizophrenia. The patient was transferred to the research metabolic unit of the Toronto Psychiatric Hospital for full investigation.

Very extensive investigations were done, the patient being maintained on a special diet under controlled conditions. Many of the tests and findings were for strictly research purposes and need not be discussed here. Some of the findings that are of general clinical interest were as follows: About every twenty-seven days, the patient lapsed suddenly into a stupor which lasted fifteen days before he emerged into a twelve-day period of relative normality. Whereas the submergence into stupor was rapid, taking place within a few hours, the emergence from stupor was much slower and more variable. Occasionally, two or three stupors would seem to be joined together in one continuous stupor. During the deep stupor of the first days, the patient would show scarcely any spontaneous activity, although he was apparently aware of his environment, reacting to it in a negative manner. In the intervening well periods, the patient would be up and around, behaving in a friendly, co-operative way.

Investigation revealed the following striking finding, typical of this type of illness, namely that physiological activity is greater at the time of stupor. The pulse rate, temperature, oxygen utilization and protein breakdown were all increased at the time of stupor. For example, the pulse rate during stupor ranged between 75 and 95 per minute with occasional peaks up to 100–120 per minute, whereas, during the well phase, the pulse rate was in the range of 60–72. While the oral temperatures during the well phase were between 97°–98.5°, they varied from 98.5° to 100.5° during the phase of stupor and even reached 102° or 103° on occasions. Oxygen utilization, as measured as the basal metabolic rate, was uniformly within the low normal range during the well phase (from −20 to −10 per cent at the onset of stupor it would rise to levels of 0 to 10 per cent. A number of other physiological findings more of interest from the research point of view also displayed a rhythmicity. These included the plasma non-protein nitrogen levels and the alpha rate of the electroencephalogram, the former increasing during the phases of stupor and the latter decreasing.

As it has been demonstrated (see references) that the administration of thyroid hormone results in the cessation of the catatonic episodes in periodic catatonia, this patient was started on triiodothyronine. The medication was administered at the beginning of a catatonic phase after the patient had been studied extensively for a period of two years during which he had experienced many cycles of catatonic and interval phases. The initial dose was 20 micrograms twice a day. The dosage was gradually raised until the basal metabolic rate was maintained in the +5 to +20 range. The catatonic state cleared at the usual time and since then the patient has appeared perfectly well, the physiological rhythms mentioned previously have disappeared, he has resumed his former employment with the telephone company and is adjusting quite satisfactorily in every respect. At the time of writing, it is now three years since the beginning of treatment with triiodothyronine. The maintenance dose for this patient is 160 micrograms a day, roughly equivalent to seven grains of desiccated thyroid daily.

Periodic catatonia is a rare type of mental disorder included under the schizophrenias. However, research workers in this field are of the opinion that the frequency of occurrence of this disorder is probably higher than is usually believed. The diagnosis of the condition evidently is often not made. Perhaps the clinician does not consider this possibility. Furthermore, because of the pressure to treat the patient as soon as possible, especially with physical measures such as electroconvulsive therapy, little opportunity is afforded to observe the cyclical nature of the disorder. The above case of catatonic stupor alternating with well phases is rather typical of one variety of periodic catatonia. The other major type is characterized by catatonic excitements alternating with well periods. If the history suggests previous episodes, then it is wise to withold any specific physical treatment and observe the patient to determine whether these disturbances follow a cyclic pattern. Each day careful note should be made of the mental status and a record kept of the rectal temperature and resting pulse rate each morning and evening. If research facilities are available, the more detailed physiological investigations referred to in the case report may aid the physician in reaching a diagnosis. If it seems definite that there are periodic episodes of catatonic illness and research facilities are not available, then a trial of thyroid medication may be undertaken. (See references for details regarding diagnosis and treatment.)

As mentioned in the introduction to this case, consideration of periodic catatonia poses some fundamental questions regarding the aetiology of the so-called functional mental illnesses. If the periodic catatonia type of schizophrenia evidently involves a physico-chemical disorder, and if apparent correction or compensation of this metabolic fault results in a return to mental health, does not this raise the possibility that other illnesses within the schizophrenic group and perhaps in the manic-depressive and other functional psychiatric groups might also be due largely to physico-chemical disturbances? Indeed there would seem to be an increasing number of psychiatrists, physiologists and biochemists who entertain such a view and who are pursuing researches in this direction. If the results of research should confirm this hypothesis, the concept of organic psychoses could conceivably be a much broader one than it is today.

REFERENCES

PRITCHARD, E. A. B.: The functional symptoms of organic disease of the brain, Lancet 268:363, Feb. 19, 1955.

SMITH, S.: Organic syndromes presenting as involutional melancholia, Brit. M.J. 2:274, July 31, 1954.

WAGGONER, R. W. and BAGCHI, B. K.: Initial masking of organic brain changes by psychic symptoms, Am. J. Psychiat. 110:904, June 1954.

GJESSING, R.: Disturbances of somatic functions in catatonia with a periodic course, and their compensation, J. Ment. Sc. 84:608, Sept. 1938.

GORNALL, A. G., EGLITIS, B., MILLER, A., STOKES, A. B. and DEWAN, J. G.: Long-term clinical and metabolic observations in periodic catatonia, Am. J. Psychiat. 109:584, Feb. 1953.

CHAPTER XV

Technical Procedures

In tabulated form are listed the tests which we have found most helpful in diagnosis. The first table outlines the simple procedures which we consider should be routine for any patient admitted to a psychiatric unit. The second table consists of those procedures from which a selection can be made once a differential diagnosis has been reached. This list is not intended to be comprehensive but should be used simply as a guide in choosing tests which may narrow down the possibilities to the correct diagnosis. In some centres different tests are used, for example, the determination of blood urea nitrogen instead of non-protein nitrogen, but the procedures listed are those with which we are familiar. Other tests, on rare occasions, may help in the diagnosis of organic psychoses, for example, the determination of the level of serum magnesium or the demonstration of "L-E" cells in a case of suspected lupus erythematosus, but these less commonly indicated tests have been omitted.

1. ROUTINE ON ALL PATIENTS

Tests	Normal results	Type of specimens
Urinalysis		
Gross appearance	Clear yellow	Freshly voided urine; catheter specimen required if patient menstruating or having vaginal discharge
Specific gravity	1.010 to 1.030	
Albumin	Negative	
Sugar	Negative	
Urobilin	Negative	
Porphyrin	Negative	
Microscopic	No casts, not more than 5 WBC/H.P.F.	
Benzidine, if any cells seen	Negative	

1. Routine on All Patients (cont'd.)

Tests	Normal results	Type of specimens
Routine blood examination Haemoglobin	Men 90–110% Women 80–100% (15.6 g. per 100 ml. = 100%)	Preferably blood from pricked ear lobe or finger; less desirable is oxalated venous blood
White blood count Blood smear	5,000–10,000 per c. mm. Normal RBC's and plate- lets Neutrophiles 60–70% Lymphocytes 20–30% Eosinophiles 1–4% Basophiles 0–0.5% Monocytes 2–6%	
Blood Wasserman	Negative	10 ml. clotted blood

2. Other Investigations*

Fields of investigation	Tests	Normal results	Type of specimens
1. Metabolic disorders (a) CARBOHYDRATE METABOLISM	Fasting blood sugar	80–120 mg. per 100 ml.	5 ml. (test tube containing oxa- late or fluoride)
	Glucose tolerance test	Normal fasting, peak lower than 160, return to fasting in 2 hrs.	
(c) PROTEIN AND AMINO ACIDS Phenylpyruvic acid excretion	Ferric chloride test†	Negative	Freshly voided urine

*Arranged in the same order as the Aetiological Classification of Organic Psychoses.

†*Test for Phenylpyruvic Acid.* If the urine is acid add a few drops of a 5% solution of ferric chloride; if phenylpyruvic acid is present, a dark green colour appears which fades away in the course of some minutes.

If the urine is alkaline, acidify slightly, preferably with dilute sulphuric acid, before adding the ferric chloride.

Alternative method: Extract the acidified urine with a small amount of ether and then pour some of the ethereal extract onto the surface of a ferric chloride solution. A dark green ring is observed at the junction of the two liquids if phenylpyruvic acid is present.

2. OTHER INVESTIGATIONS (*cont'd.*)

Fields of investigation	Tests	Normal results	Type of specimens
(*d*) VITAMIN DEFICIENCY			
(i) Thiamine	Pyruvic acid levels, fasting and after glucose	This investigation requires special laboratory facilities; the directors of local laboratories should be consulted	
(iii) Vitamin B12 deficiency	Blood smear		
	Red blood count	Men 4.5–6 million/c.mm. Women 4.5–5.4 million/c.mm.	Blood from pricked ear lobe or finger
	Haemoglobin Haematocrit	Men 41–52 Women 38–46	Oxalated venous blood 5 ml.
	Histamine test meal		Gastric contents
(*e*) MINERALS			
(i) Iron deficiency	Haemoglobin Blood smear Stool benzidine	Negative	Fresh stool
(ii) and (iii) Calcium deficiency and excess	Serum calcium	9–11 mg. per 100 ml.	10 ml. clotted blood
	Serum phosphorus	3–4.5 mg. per 100 ml.	5 ml. clotted blood
	Alkaline phosphatase	3–13 Kay-Jenner units	5 ml. clotted blood
(iv) Disordered copper metabolism	Copper excretion	This investigation requires special procedures; the directors of local laboratories should be consulted	
(*f*) PORPHYRINS	Tests for porphyrins*	Negative	Urine

Tests for Porphyrins. Voided urine may be normal in colour or a shade varying from pink to port-wine. If the urine is normal in colour, test with litmus paper, and if it is not acid add a few drops of acetic acid until the urine is acid. Then tape the test-tube of urine to a window in the sunlight. The pink to port-wine colour may appear gradually. Failure of the colour to develop does not exclude porphyrinuria.

A more specific test is as follows:

(1) 2 ml. each of urine and Ehrlich's reagent are mixed in a test-tube,

(2) 4 ml. of a saturated solution of sodium acetate is added to the above mixture,

(3) 2 ml. of chloroform is then added and the tube is shaken,

(4) The persistence of a rich Burgundy tint in the supernatant aqueous fraction is indicative of a positive reaction for porphobilinogen.

2. OTHER INVESTIGATIONS (*cont'd.*)

Fields of investigation	Tests	Normal results	Type of specimens
(*g*) ELECTROLYTES	Serum sodium	310–338 mg. per 100 ml. or 135–147 mEq/l	10 ml. clotted blood
	Potassium	16–22 mg. per 100 ml. or 4–5.5 mEq/l	10 ml. separated serum†
	Chloride (as NaCl)	580–620 mg. per 100 ml. or 99–108 mEq/l	10 ml. clotted blood
(*h*) ACID BASE BALANCE	CO₂ combining power	55–75 vols. per 100 ml. or 24–33 mEq/l	10 ml. oxalated blood
(*i*) WATER	Haemoglobin	Men 90–110% Women 80–100% (15.6 g. = 100%)	Preferably blood from pricked ear lobe or finger; less desirable is oxalated venous blood
	Haematocrit	Men 41–52 Women 38–46	5 ml. oxalated venous blood
	Measured fluid intake and output	Fluid intake over 1500 ml. Urine output over 1000 ml.	
	N.P.N.	25–40 mg. per 100 ml.	10 ml. oxalated blood
(*j*) HORMONES (i) Pituitary	B.M.R.	−15 to +10 per cent	
	Eosinophile count	100–450 per c. mm.	Blood from pricked ear lobe or finger
	Tests for functions of target organs, e.g., thyroid, adrenal, gonads		
	17-ketosteroids	Men 10–20 mg./24 hr. Women 6-17 mg./24 hr.	24 hr. urine collection packed in ice
	Glucocorticoids	3-10 mg./24 hr.	

†Spun and separated right away.

2. OTHER INVESTIGATIONS (*cont'd.*)

Fields of investigation	Tests	Normal results	Type of specimens
(ii) Adrenal cortical function	Eosinophile count ACTH test* Serum electrolytes (see previous page) Fasting blood sugar. Glucose tolerance test	100–450/c. mm. Eosinophiles fall more than 50% by end of 4 hrs.	Blood from pricked ear lobe or finger
(iii) Thyroid function	BMR Protein-bound iodine Radio active iodine uptake	−15 to +10 per cent 4–8 microg. per 100 ml. 10–40% in 24 hrs.	10 ml. clotted blood

(iv) Parathyroid: See under calcium deficiency and excess, 1 (*e*) (ii) and (iii)

(v) Pancreas: See under carbohydrate metabolism 1 (*a*).

(*k*) OXYGEN			
Carbon monoxide poisoning	Spectroscopic blood examination	Negative	Consult local laboratory
2. Disordered blood supply 3. Mechanical stresses 4. Infections 6. Degenerations	C.S.F. examination	Pressure: 60–150 mm. H₂O (horizontal position) clear, aqueous Cells: less than 5 per c. mm. Protein: less than 40 mg. per 100 ml. W.R.: negative.	C.S.F. 15 ml.

*ACTH tests. (1) Do an eosinophile count. Give 25 mg. of ACTH, i.m.; four hours later do another eosinophile count. A failure of the count to fall 50% indicates hypofunction of the adrenal cortices. This test is best begun about noon because there is normally a spontaneous morning fall in the eosinophile count which may exceed 50%.
(2) A much more reliable procedure is the forty-eight hour ACTH test. This investigation requires special laboratory facilities. For further information consult the directors of your local laboratories.

2. OTHER INVESTIGATIONS (*cont'd.*)

Fields of investigation	Tests	Normal results	Type of specimens
		Colloidal gold readings of 1111111111 or less. Chloride: 700–750 mg. per 100 ml. Sugar: 50–80 mg./ 100 ml. Culture: negative Pandy: negative or weakly positive	
4. Infections	Blood cultures	Negative	Sterile oxalated blood
	Agglutination tests for typhoid, paratyphoid brucella	Negative	Clotted blood
	Agglutination tests for typhus and viruses	Negative	Clotted blood
	Heterophile antibody test	Negative	Clotted blood
	Cultures of sputa, discharges, stool, urine	Negative	Fresh material
	Tuberculin test 1/20 mg. initially	Negative or a raised erythema less than 1 cm. at 48 hrs.	
5. Intoxications (*a*) EXOGENOUS	Bromide	Negative	10 ml. clotted blood
	Barbiturates	Negative	35 ml. oxalated blood
	Morphine	Negative	24 hr. urine collection
	Sulphas	Negative	5 ml. blood in test-tube containing fluoride
	Mercury	Negative	24 hr. urine collection
	Thiocyanate	Negative	5 ml. clotted blood
	Alcohol	Negative	5 ml. clotted blood

2. OTHER INVESTIGATIONS (*cont'd.*)

Fields of investigation	Tests	Normal results	Type of specimens
	Lead	Negative	24 hr. urine collection
	Manganese	Negative	24 hr. urine collection
	Arsenic	Negative	24 hr. urine collection
(*b*) ENDOGENOUS			
Kidney function	N.P.N.	25–40 mg. per 100 ml.	10 ml. oxalated blood
	Mosenthal 2 hr. test		
Liver function	van den Bergh	0.1–1.0 mg. per 100 ml. (indirect)	5 ml. clotted blood
	Cephalin cholesterol flocculation	Negative	5 ml. clotted blood
	Serum proteins	6–8 g. per 100 ml. Albumin 3.5–5.5 g. Globulin 1.5–3.0 g.	10 ml. clotted blood
	Bromsulphthalein	Less than 5% retention at 45 minutes	5 ml. clotted blood
	Alkaline phosphatase	3–13 Kay-Jenner units	5 ml. clotted blood
	Urine urobilin	Negative	Fresh urine specimen
6. Degenerations	C.S.F. examination Air encephalogram Electroencephalo-gram Psychological tests		
7. Paroxysmal cerebral dysrhythmia	Electroencephalo-gram		

GENERAL AND MISCELLANEOUS REFERENCES

In this manual many topics are mentioned so briefly that comprehensive texts should be consulted when diagnostic and other difficulties arise. We have found the following text-books of great value:

BRAIN, W. R.: Diseases of the Nervous System, ed. 5, Toronto, Oxford Medical Publications, 1955.

HARRISON, T. R.: Principles of Internal Medicine, ed. 2, Philadelphia, The Blakiston Co., 1954.

HENDERSON, D. K. and GILLESPIE, R. D.: A Textbook of Psychiatry, ed. 8, Toronto, Oxford University Press, 1956.

NOYES, A. P.: Modern Clinical Psychiatry, ed. 4, Philadelphia, W. B. Saunders Co., 1953.

The following articles are of interest. They are included here because they do not fit readily into the other lists of references:

CHARATAN, F. B. and BRIERLEY, J. B.: Mental disorder associated with primary lung carcinoma, Brit. M.J. 1:765, April 7, 1956.

GALLINEK, A.: Syndrome of episodes of hypersomnia, bulimia and abnormal mental states, J.A.M.A. 154:1081, March 27, 1954.

HÖÖK, O.: Sarcoidosis with involvement of the nervous system. Report of nine cases, Arch. Neurol. & Psychiat. 71:554, May 1954.

INDEX

Lightning Source UK Ltd.
Milton Keynes UK
UKHW010013210722
406167UK00002B/463